About the Author

Louise Pearce is a wife, a mother of three children, and a grandmother to four. Throughout her life, she has been actively involved with her family and their activities while developing her creative talents in jewelry design and in spiritual writing. She is an enthusiastic person who loves to try anything new and different, undaunted by the how or the when. With great energy, she can take a leap into the unknown with energy to reinvent herself and take up new challenges. She resides in Sherwood Park with her husband, Bob, who is retired and active in fitness, gardening, and travel.

Louise Pearce

You Got This

A Journal to Mental Wellness

MACAULEY PUBLISHERS®

CAMBRIDGE • NEW YORK • SHARJAH

Ordering Information

Quantity sales: Special discounts are available on quantity purchases by corporations, associations, and others. For details, contact the publisher at the address below.

Publisher's Cataloging-in-Publication data

Pearce, Louise

You Got This

ISBN 9798897892389 (Paperback)

ISBN 9798897892396 (ePub e-book)

Library of Congress Control Number: 2025927701

www.austinmacauleyusa.com

First Published 2026

Austin Macauley Publishers LLC

40 Wall Street, 33rd Floor, Suite 3302

New York, NY 10005

USA

mail-usa@austinmacauley.com

+1 (646) 5125767

Acknowledgments

Once again, I thank my sister Adele Perrett for her unfailing patience and guidance in putting this book together.

Introduction

As we continue our journey to our own mental wellness, we look back and understand how far we have come and what we have accomplished. Although we still have work to do and goals to meet, we must believe that the important thing is the effort we put in to reach these goals.

This effort will change and improve each and every one of us as we venture forth with confidence and perseverance.
Let's continue.

I am cared for; I am loved

I am intelligent; I am talented

I am accomplished; I am appreciated

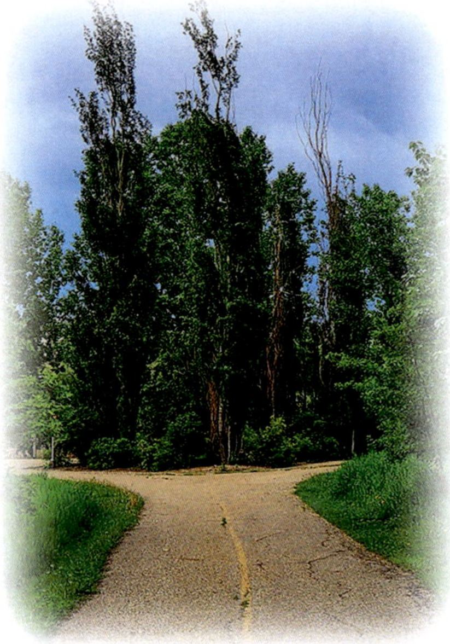

T-Shirt Thought

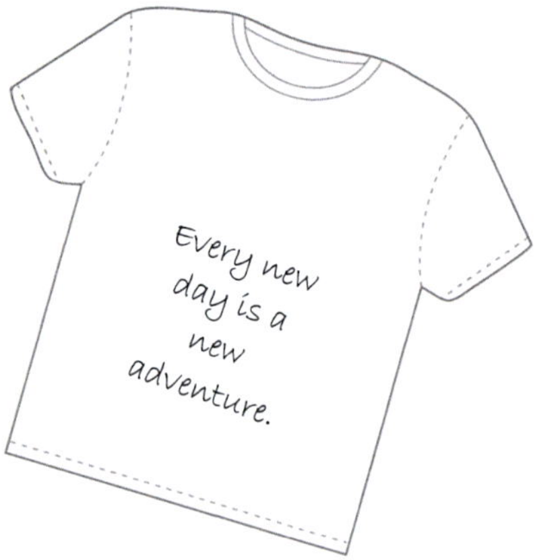

I am grateful; I am sympathetic

I am understanding; I am positive everyday

I am strong; I am dependable

I am honest; I am trustworthy

I will express my gratitude to the universe every day for all that I have and all that I am.

End of Day

In every imperfect day, we can find a little perfection.

CONTEMPLATION

I am cared for; I am loved

I am intelligent; I am talented

I am accomplished; I am appreciated

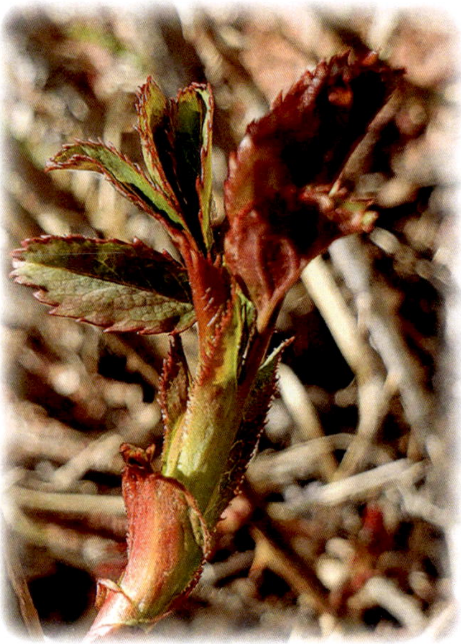

T-Shirt Thought

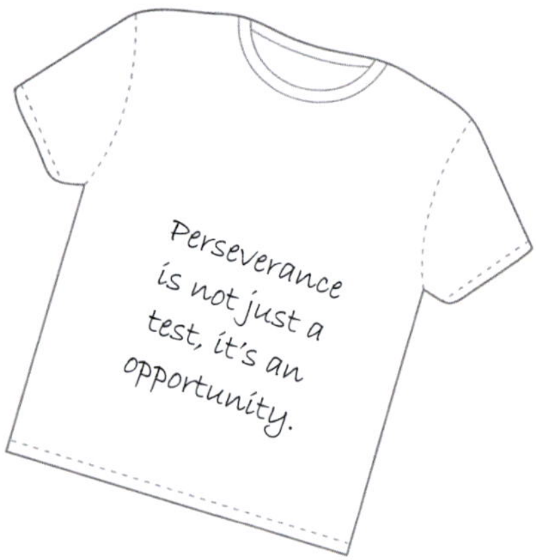

I am grateful; I am sympathetic

I am understanding; I am positive everyday

I am strong; I am dependable

I am honest; I am trustworthy

I will express my gratitude to the universe every day for all that I have and all that I am.

End of Day

Becoming stronger is hard, worthy work. Do it every day.

CONTEMPLATION

I am cared for; I am loved

I am intelligent; I am talented

I am accomplished; I am appreciated

T-Shirt Thought

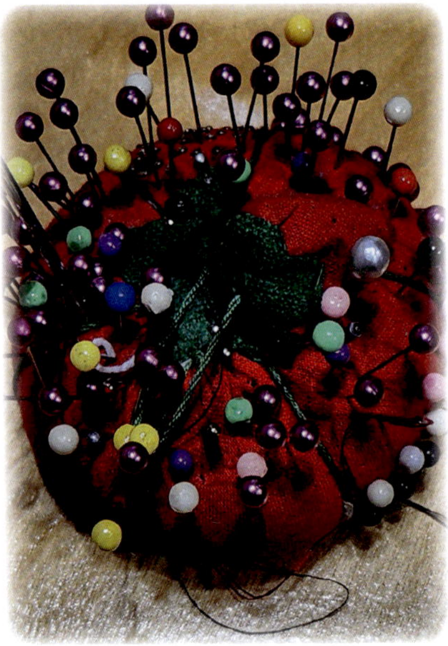

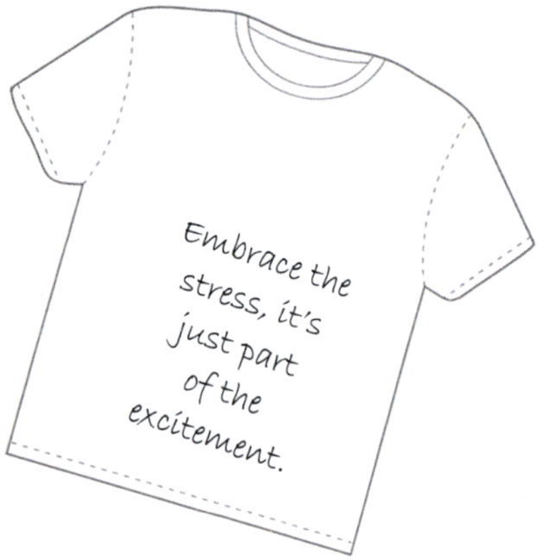

I am grateful; I am sympathetic

I am understanding; I am positive everyday

I am strong; I am dependable

I am honest; I am trustworthy

I will express my gratitude to the universe every day for all that I have and all that I am.

End of Day

No matter what happens, life will go on, so relax and ride the wave.

CONTEMPLATION

I am cared for; I am loved

I am intelligent; I am talented

I am accomplished; I am appreciated

T-Shirt Thought

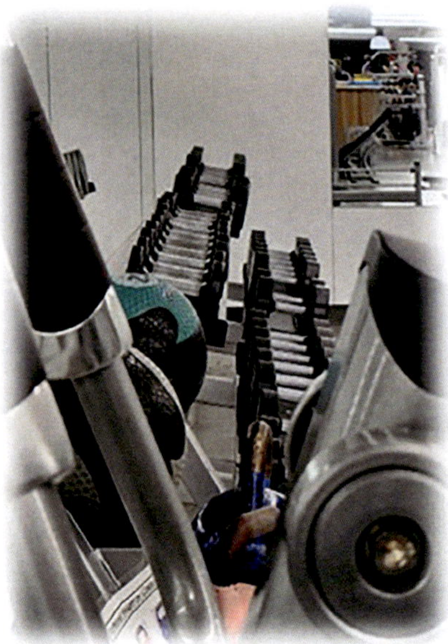

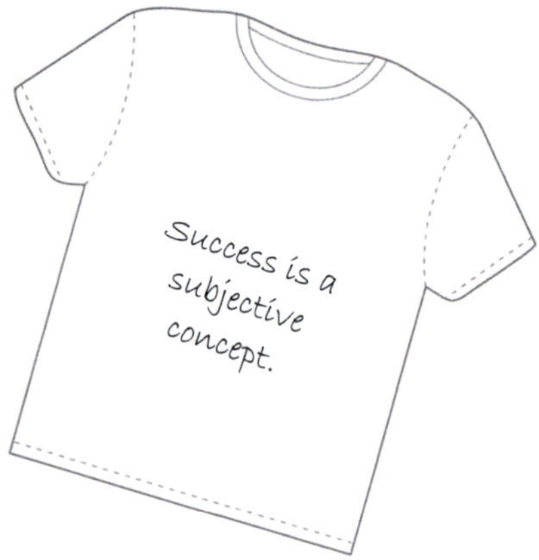

I am grateful; I am sympathetic

I am understanding; I am positive everyday

I am strong; I am dependable

I am honest; I am trustworthy

I will express my gratitude to the universe every day for all that I have and all that I am.

End of Day

A good attitude and a good workout equal a great day.

CONTEMPLATION

I am cared for; I am loved

I am intelligent; I am talented

I am accomplished; I am appreciated

T-Shirt Thought

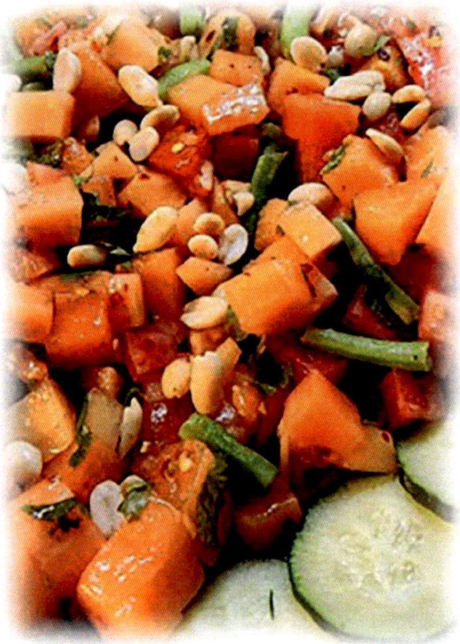

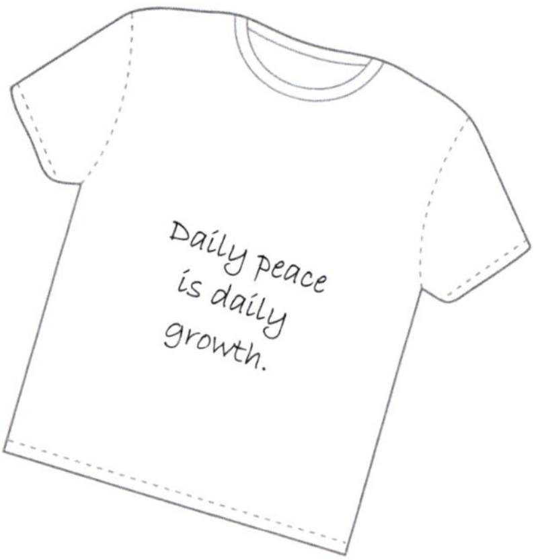

I am grateful; I am sympathetic

I am understanding; I am positive everyday

I am strong; I am dependable

I am honest; I am trustworthy

I will express my gratitude to the universe every day for all that I have and all that I am.

End of Day

Playing with happy colored flowers always picks me up on a down day.

CONTEMPLATION

I am cared for; I am loved

I am intelligent; I am talented

I am accomplished; I am appreciated

T-Shirt Thought

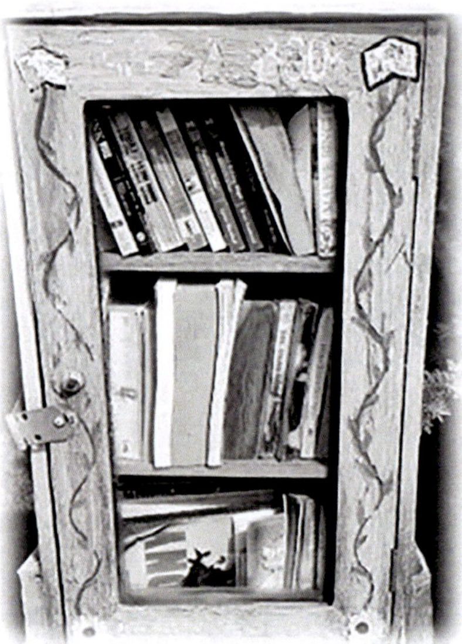

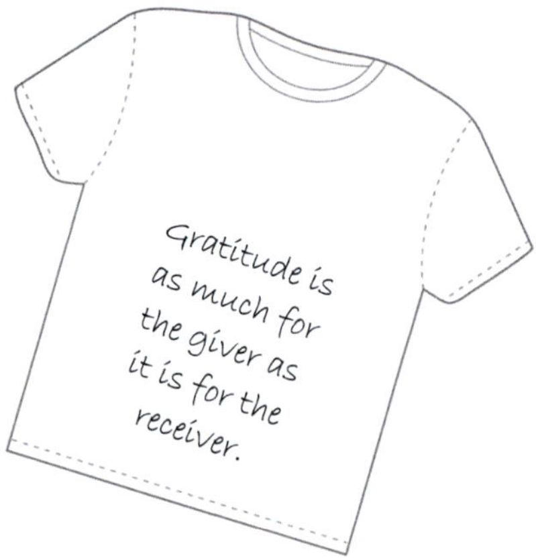

I am grateful; I am sympathetic

I am understanding; I am positive everyday

I am strong; I am dependable

I am honest; I am trustworthy

I will express my gratitude to the universe every day for all that I have and all that I am.

End of Day

A few creative moments can put a smile on the faces of so many.

CONTEMPLATION

TOGETHER ON THE PATH

I am cared for; I am loved

I am intelligent; I am talented

I am accomplished; I am appreciated

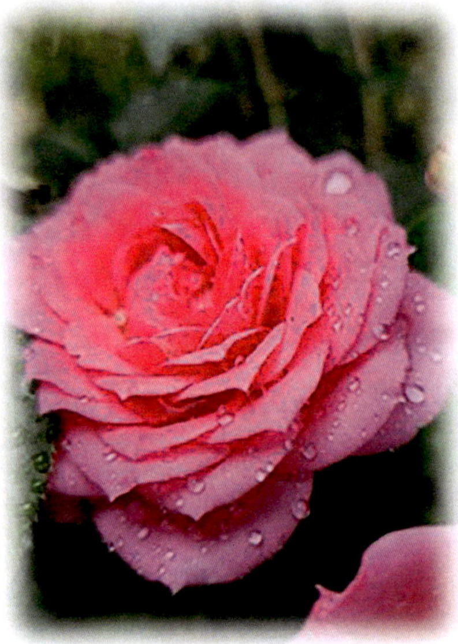

T-Shirt Thought

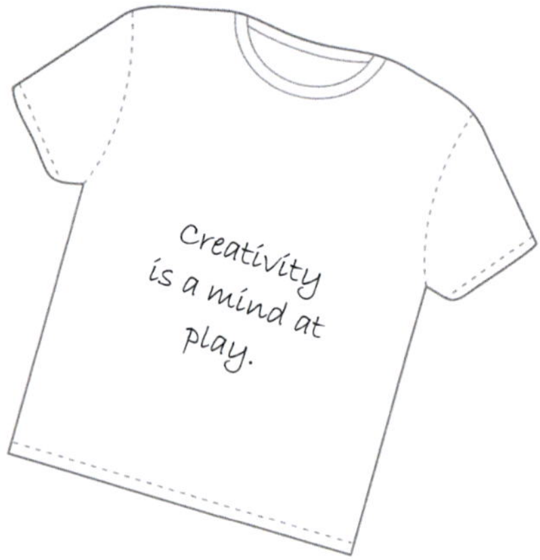

I am grateful; I am sympathetic

I am understanding; I am positive everyday

I am strong; I am dependable

I am honest; I am trustworthy

I will express my gratitude to the universe every day for all that I have and all that I am.

End of Day

Be someone's hero, every chance you get.

CONTEMPLATION

TOGETHER ON THE PATH

I am cared for; I am loved

I am intelligent; I am talented

I am accomplished; I am appreciated

T-Shirt Thought

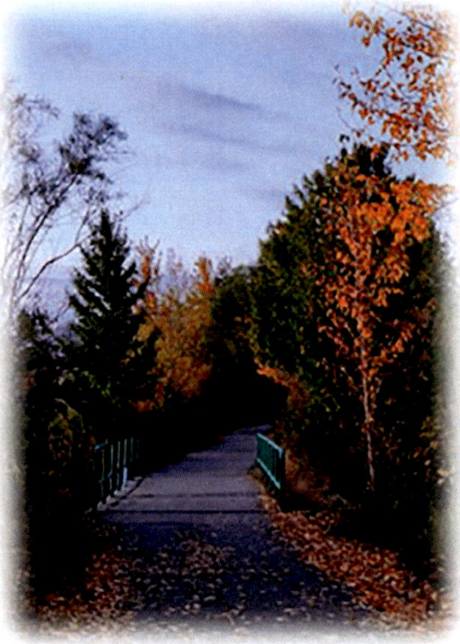

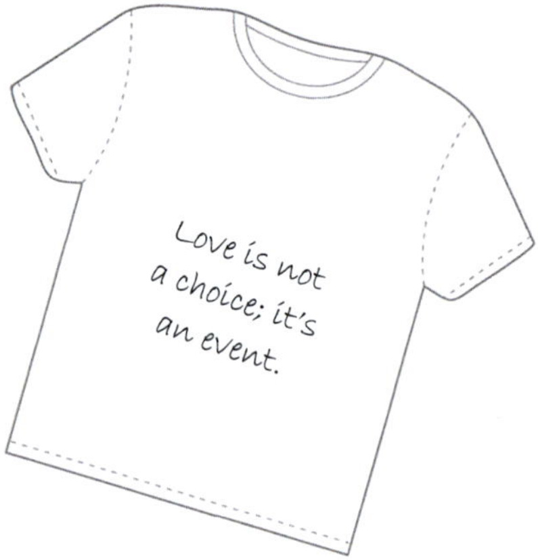

I am grateful; I am sympathetic

I am understanding; I am positive everyday

I am strong; I am dependable

I am honest; I am trustworthy

I will express my gratitude to the universe every day for all that I have and all that I am.

End of Day

Love given and love taken is a true daily treasure, one not to be taken for granted.

CONTEMPLATION

I am cared for; I am loved

I am intelligent; I am talented

I am accomplished; I am appreciated

T-Shirt Thought

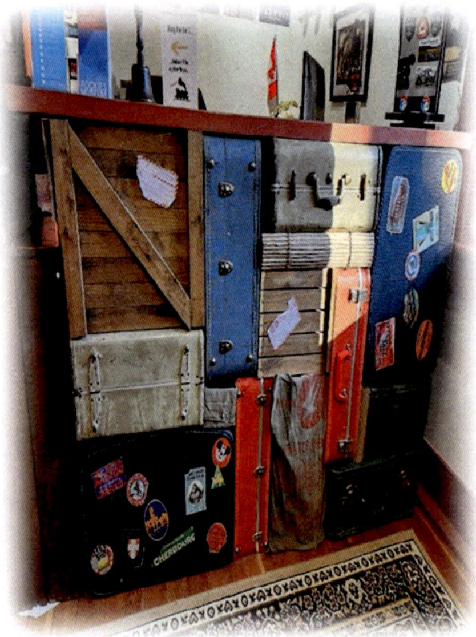

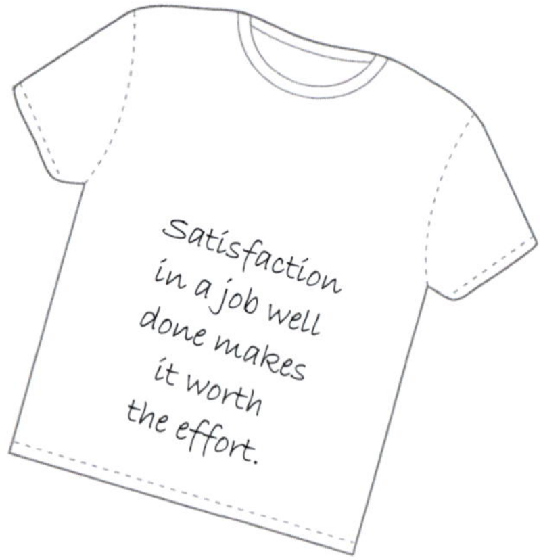

I am grateful; I am sympathetic

I am understanding; I am positive everyday

I am strong; I am dependable

I am honest; I am trustworthy

I will express my gratitude to the universe every day for all that I have and all that I am.

End of Day

It feels so gratifying to have your work visually confirmed and appreciated.

CONTEMPLATION

I am cared for; I am loved

I am intelligent; I am talented

I am accomplished; I am appreciated

T-Shirt Thought

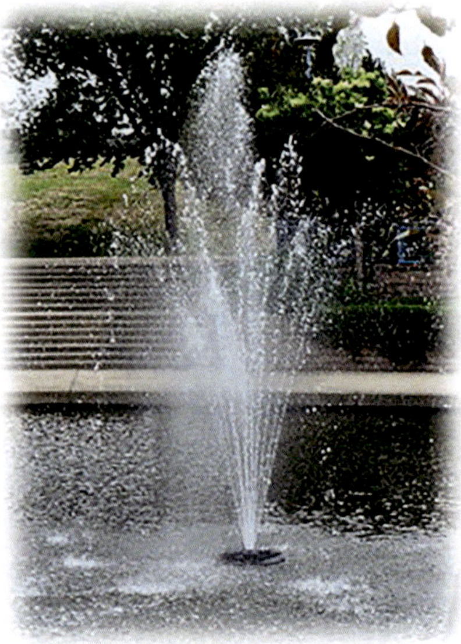

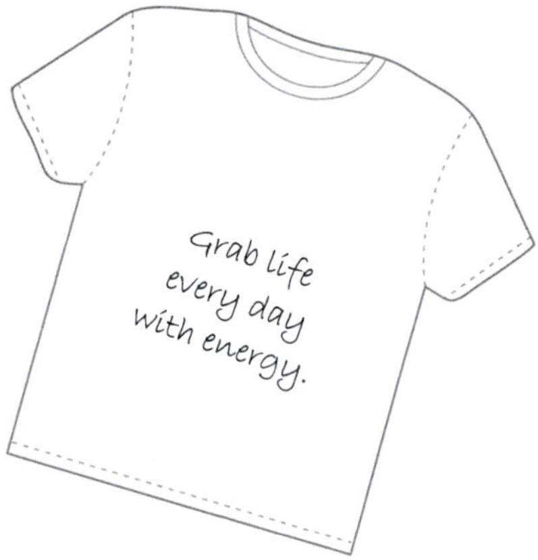

I am grateful; I am sympathetic

I am understanding; I am positive everyday

I am strong; I am dependable

I am honest; I am trustworthy

I will express my gratitude to the universe every day for all that I have and all that I am.

End of Day

To pump up your enthusiasm, just change your perspective and, your activity... MOVE.

CONTEMPLATION

I am cared for; I am loved

I am intelligent; I am talented

I am accomplished; I am appreciated

T-Shirt Thought

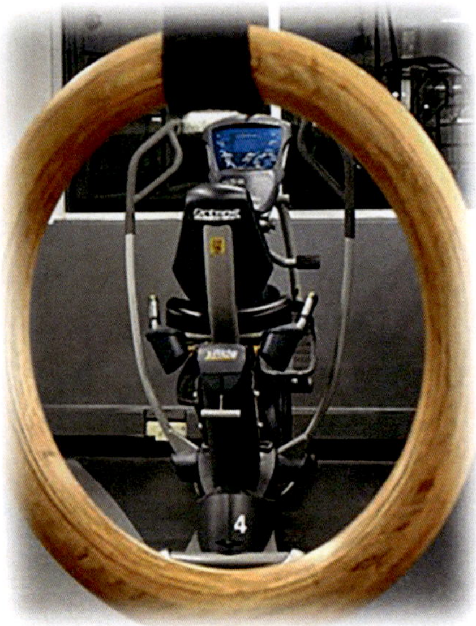

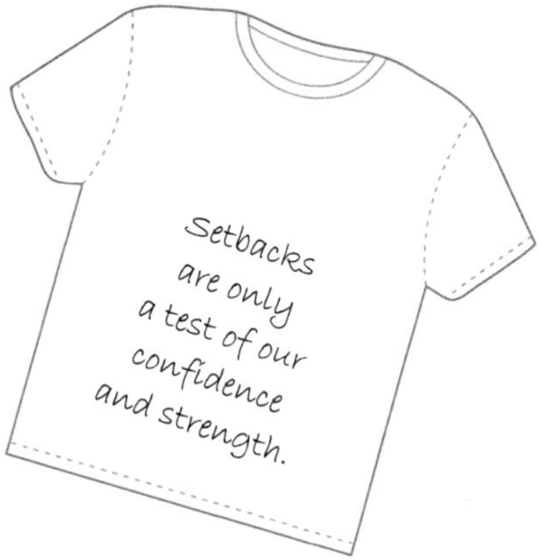

I am grateful; I am sympathetic

I am understanding; I am positive everyday

I am strong; I am dependable

I am honest; I am trustworthy

I will express my gratitude to the universe every day for all that I have and all that I am.

End of Day

Rewards for work well done are confirmations of the work itself.

CONTEMPLATION

I am cared for; I am loved

I am intelligent; I am talented

I am accomplished; I am appreciated

T-Shirt Thought

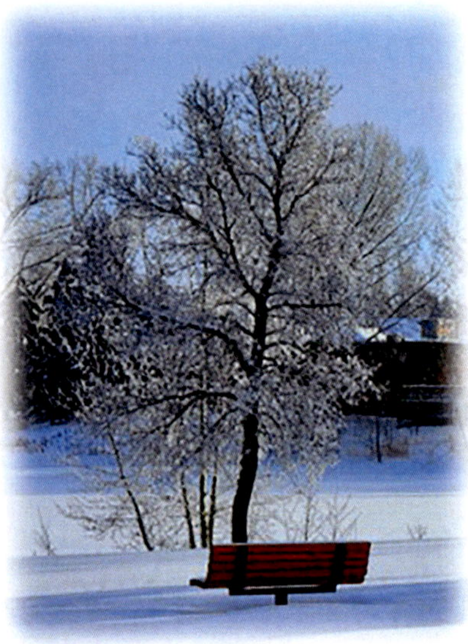

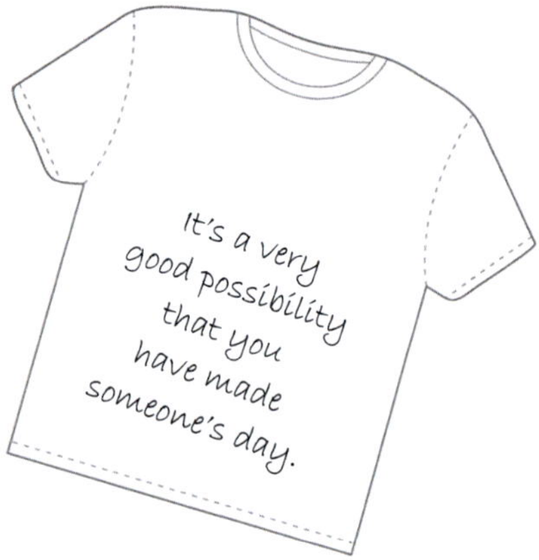

I am grateful; I am sympathetic

I am understanding; I am positive everyday

I am strong; I am dependable

I am honest; I am trustworthy

I will express my gratitude to the universe every day for all that I have and all that I am.

End of Day

When the struggles of the day seem endless, just power through with the confidence you know you have.

CONTEMPLATION

I am cared for; I am loved

I am intelligent; I am talented

I am accomplished; I am appreciated

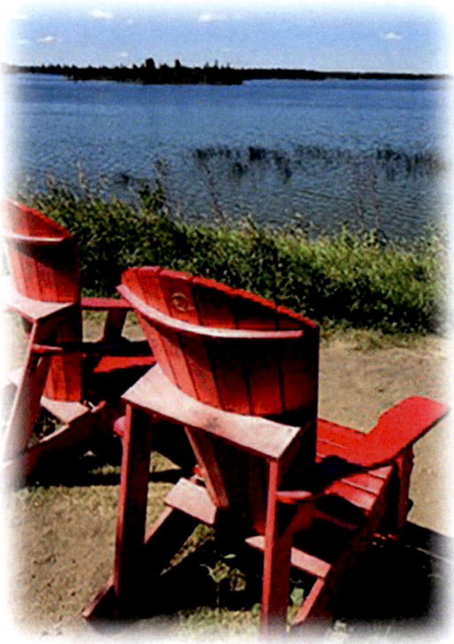

T-Shirt Thought

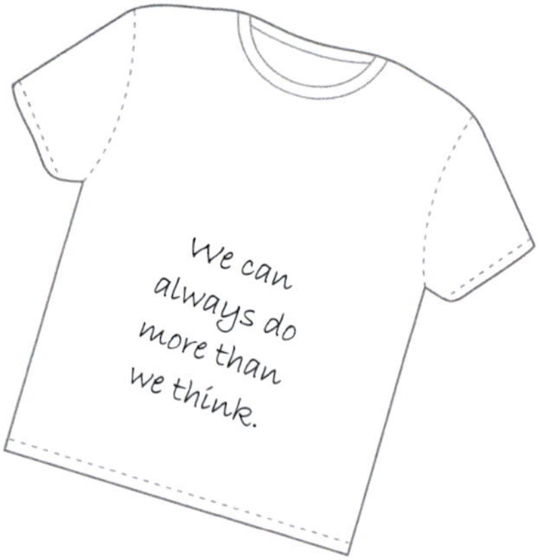

I am grateful; I am sympathetic

I am understanding; I am positive everyday

I am strong; I am dependable

I am honest; I am trustworthy

I will express my gratitude to the universe every day for all that I have and all that I am.

End of Day

Every challenge makes us stronger, more confident, and more powerful.

CONTEMPLATION

TOGETHER ON THE PATH

I am cared for; I am loved

I am intelligent; I am talented

I am accomplished; I am appreciated

T-Shirt Thought

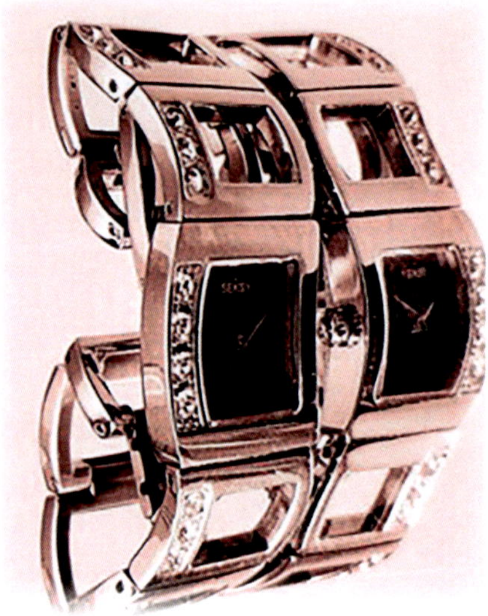

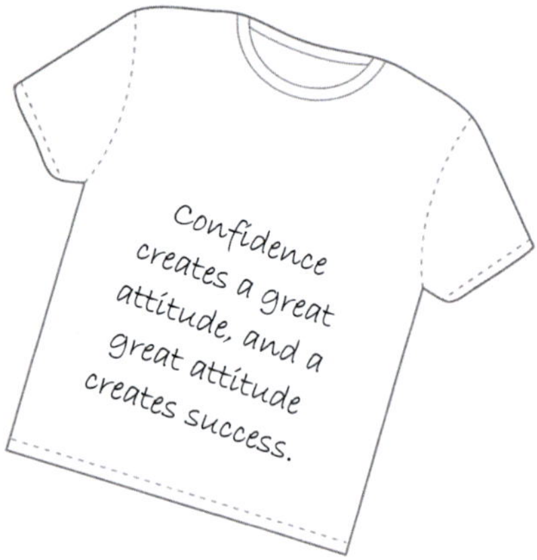

I am grateful; I am sympathetic

I am understanding; I am positive everyday

I am strong; I am dependable

I am honest; I am trustworthy

I will express my gratitude to the universe every day for all that I have and all that I am.

End of Day

When someone appreciates your work, your heart soars.

CONTEMPLATION

TOGETHER ON THE PATH

I am cared for; I am loved

I am intelligent; I am talented

I am accomplished; I am appreciated

T-Shirt Thought

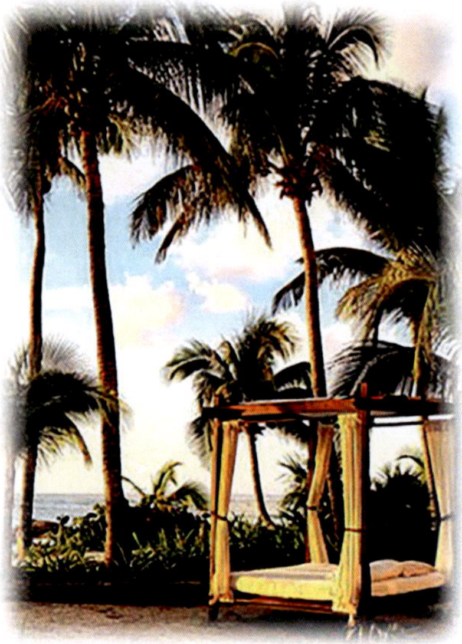

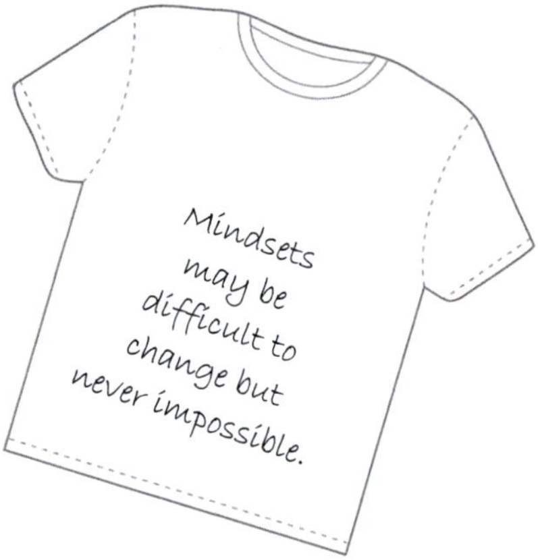

I am grateful; I am sympathetic

I am understanding; I am positive everyday

I am strong; I am dependable

I am honest; I am trustworthy

I will express my gratitude to the universe every day for all that I have and all that I am.

End of Day

Sometimes it's difficult to see the positive but it's always, always there.

CONTEMPLATION

TOGETHER ON THE PATH

I am cared for; I am loved

I am intelligent; I am talented

I am accomplished; I am appreciated

T-Shirt Thought

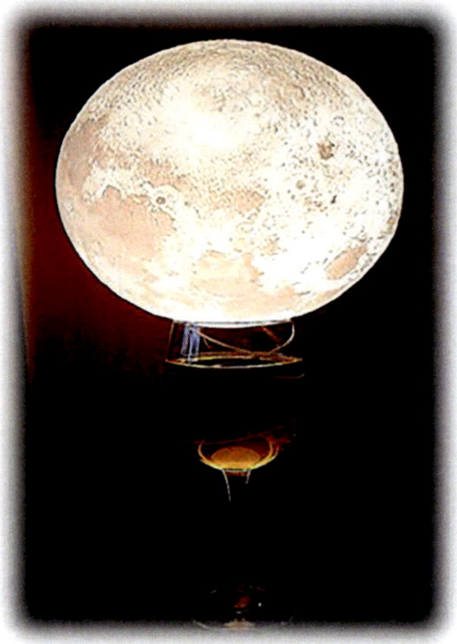

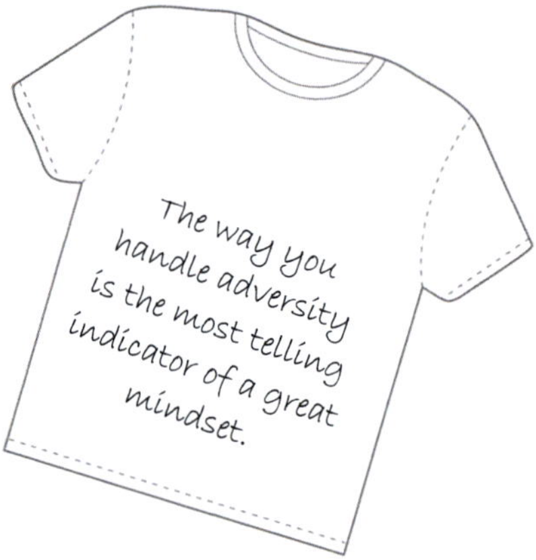

I am grateful; I am sympathetic

I am understanding; I am positive everyday

I am strong; I am dependable

I am honest; I am trustworthy

I will express my gratitude to the universe every day for all that I have and all that I am.

End of Day

Perseverance through stress and exhaustion is twice as sweet.

CONTEMPLATION

I am cared for; I am loved

I am intelligent; I am talented

I am accomplished; I am appreciated

T-Shirt Thought

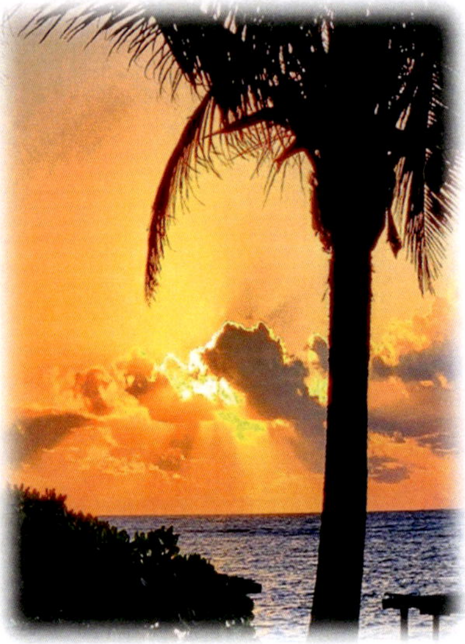

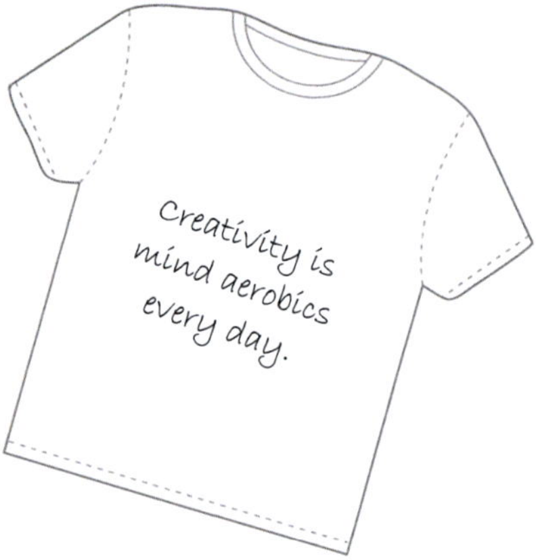

I am grateful; I am sympathetic

I am understanding; I am positive everyday

I am strong; I am dependable

I am honest; I am trustworthy

I will express my gratitude to the universe every day for all that I have and all that I am.

End of Day

Accepting a new photography challenge is always exciting, always energizing.

CONTEMPLATION

I am cared for; I am loved

I am intelligent; I am talented

I am accomplished; I am appreciated

T-Shirt Thought

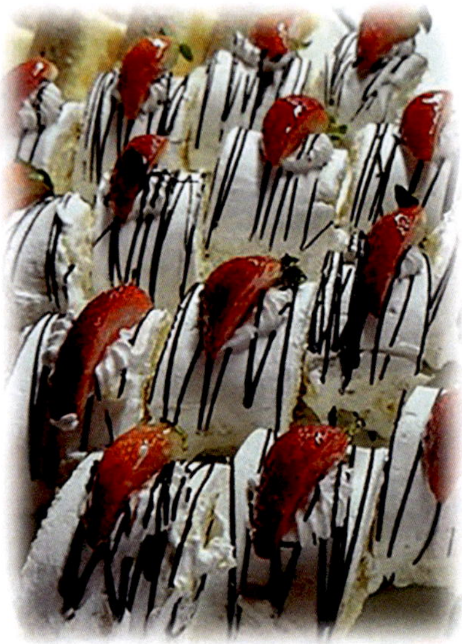

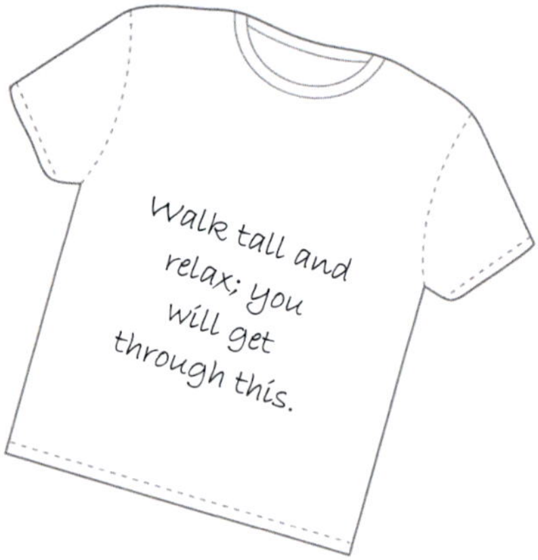

I am grateful; I am sympathetic

I am understanding; I am positive everyday

I am strong; I am dependable

I am honest; I am trustworthy

I will express my gratitude to the universe every day for all that I have and all that I am.

End of Day

Walking tall every day is not always easy, but it is ALWAYS rewarding.

CONTEMPLATION

I am cared for; I am loved

I am intelligent; I am talented

I am accomplished; I am appreciated

T-Shirt Thought

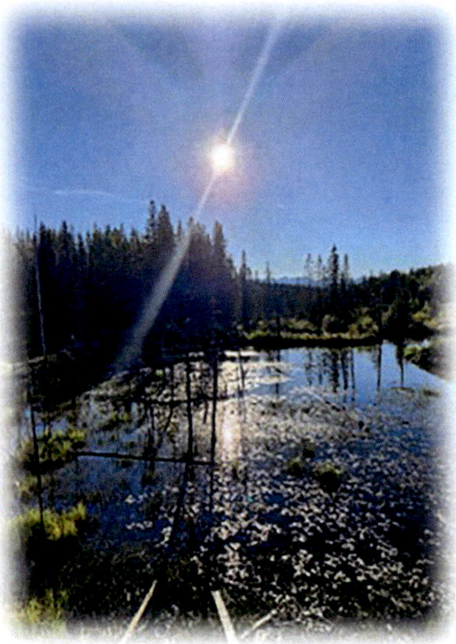

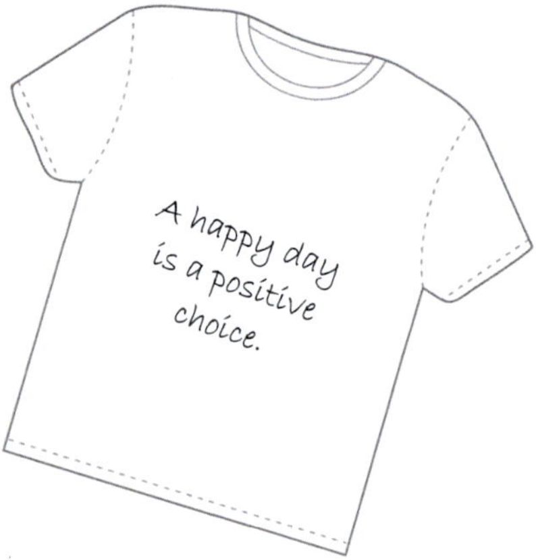

I am grateful; I am sympathetic

I am understanding; I am positive everyday

I am strong; I am dependable

I am honest; I am trustworthy

I will express my gratitude to the universe every day for all that I have and all that I am.

End of Day

Surround yourself with happy people every day. It will energize you every time.

CONTEMPLATION

I am cared for; I am loved

I am intelligent; I am talented

I am accomplished; I am appreciated

T-Shirt Thought

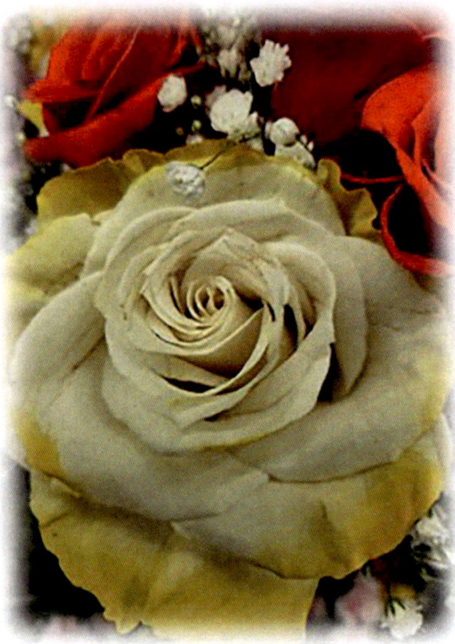

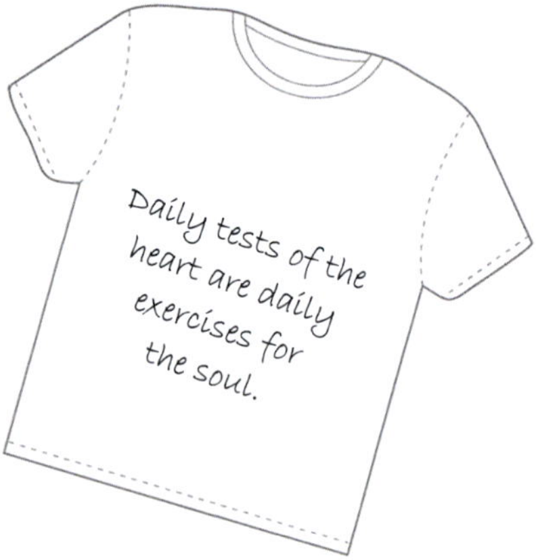

I am grateful; I am sympathetic

I am understanding; I am positive everyday

I am strong; I am dependable

I am honest; I am trustworthy

I will express my gratitude to the universe every day for all that I have and all that I am.

End of Day

Crying during a good movie does not make me weak, it just makes me more connected to life.

CONTEMPLATION

I am cared for; I am loved

I am intelligent; I am talented

I am accomplished; I am appreciated

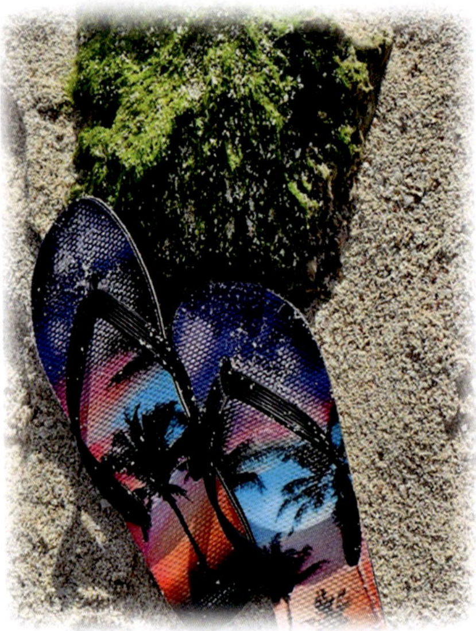

T-Shirt Thought

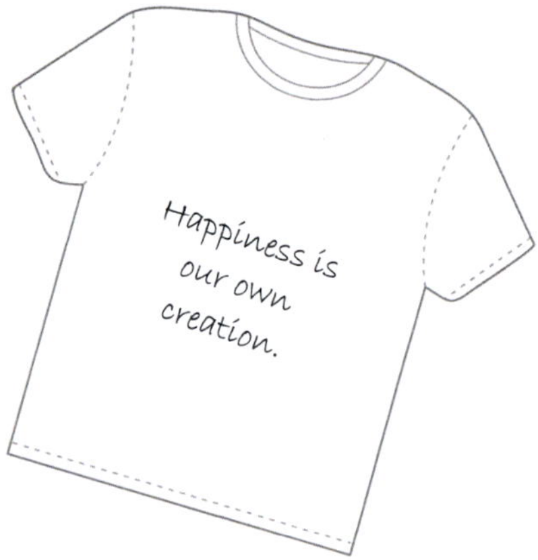

I am grateful; I am sympathetic

I am understanding; I am positive everyday

I am strong; I am dependable

I am honest; I am trustworthy

I will express my gratitude to the universe every day for all that I have and all that I am.

End of Day

A gorgeous sunny day can lighten up my soul every time.

CONTEMPLATION

TOGETHER ON THE PATH

I am cared for; I am loved

I am intelligent; I am talented

I am accomplished; I am appreciated

T-Shirt Thought

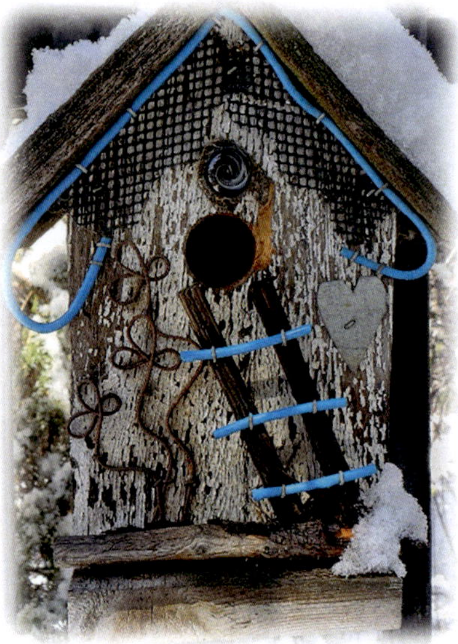

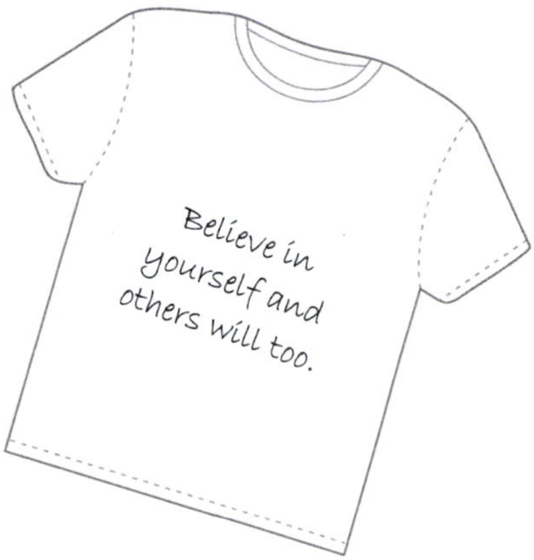

I am grateful; I am sympathetic

I am understanding; I am positive everyday

I am strong; I am dependable

I am honest; I am trustworthy

I will express my gratitude to the universe every day for all that I have and all that I am.

End of Day

Look back on your successes so you can look ahead to more.

CONTEMPLATION

TOGETHER ON THE PATH

I am cared for; I am loved

I am intelligent; I am talented

I am accomplished; I am appreciated

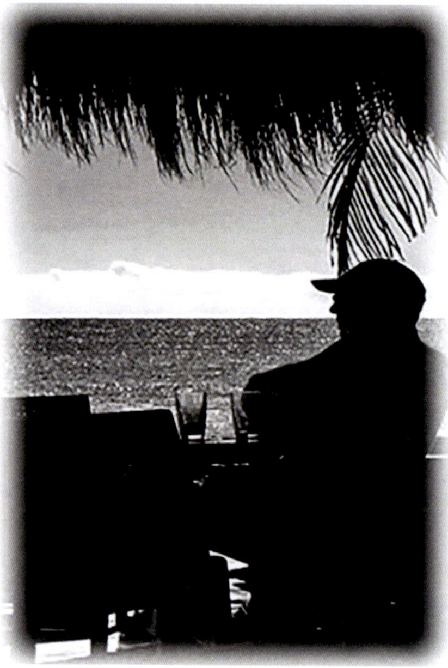

T-Shirt Thought

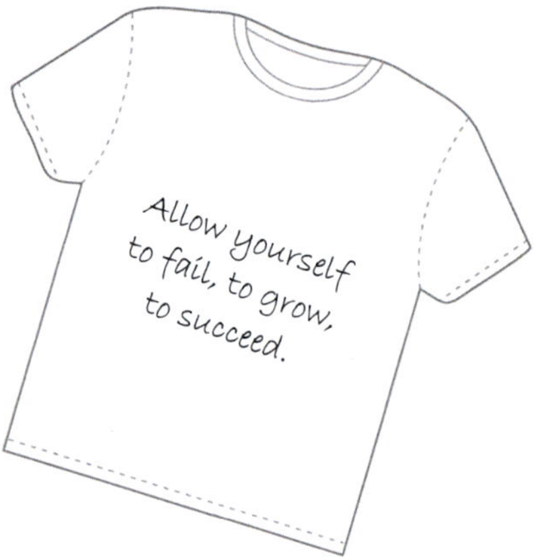

I am grateful; I am sympathetic

I am understanding; I am positive everyday

I am strong; I am dependable

I am honest; I am trustworthy

I will express my gratitude to the universe every day for all that I have and all that I am.

End of Day

Having the confidence to improve my daily mindset is the most peaceful feeling.

CONTEMPLATION

TOGETHER ON THE PATH

I am cared for; I am loved

I am intelligent; I am talented

I am accomplished; I am appreciated

T-Shirt Thought

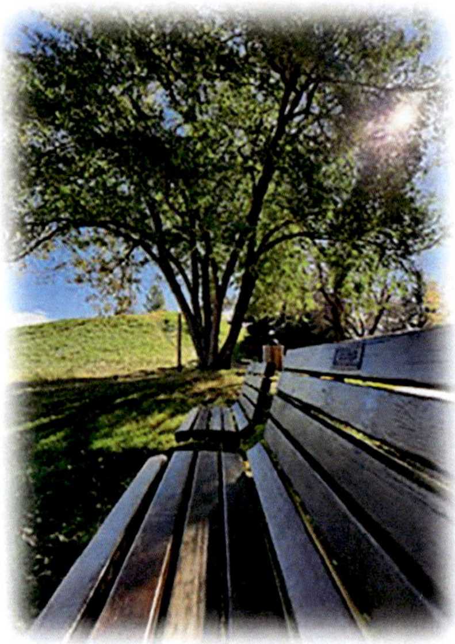

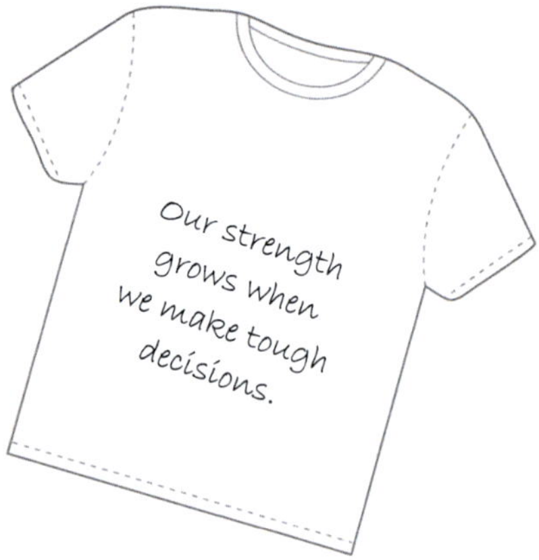

I am grateful; I am sympathetic

I am understanding; I am positive everyday

I am strong; I am dependable

I am honest; I am trustworthy

I will express my gratitude to the universe every day for all that I have and all that I am.

End of Day

Self-motivation must come from within every day.

CONTEMPLATION

I am cared for; I am loved

I am intelligent; I am talented

I am accomplished; I am appreciated

T-Shirt Thought

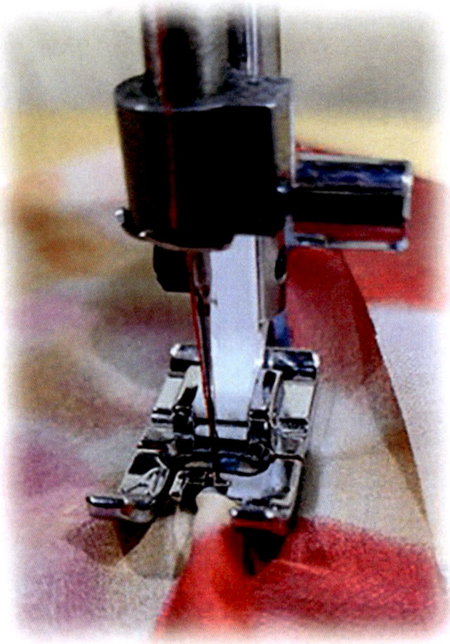

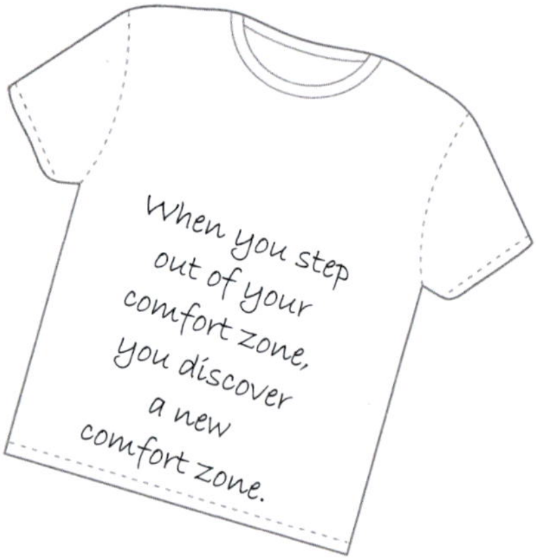

I am grateful; I am sympathetic

I am understanding; I am positive everyday

I am strong; I am dependable

I am honest; I am trustworthy

I will express my gratitude to the universe every day for all that I have and all that I am.

End of Day

When you are reminded of your value to others, it rejuvenates your soul.

CONTEMPLATION

TOGETHER ON THE PATH

I am cared for; I am loved

I am intelligent; I am talented

I am accomplished; I am appreciated

T-Shirt Thought

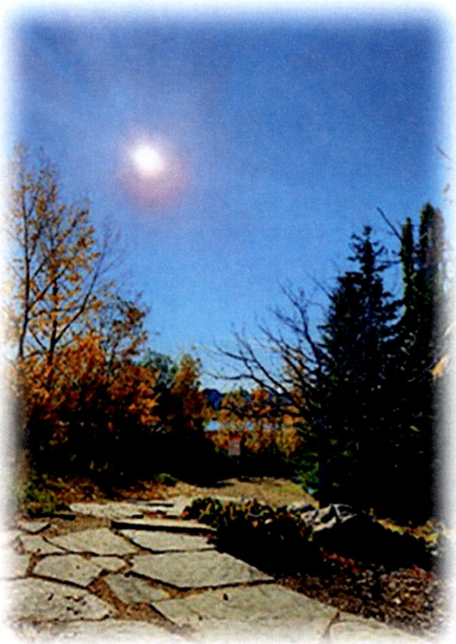

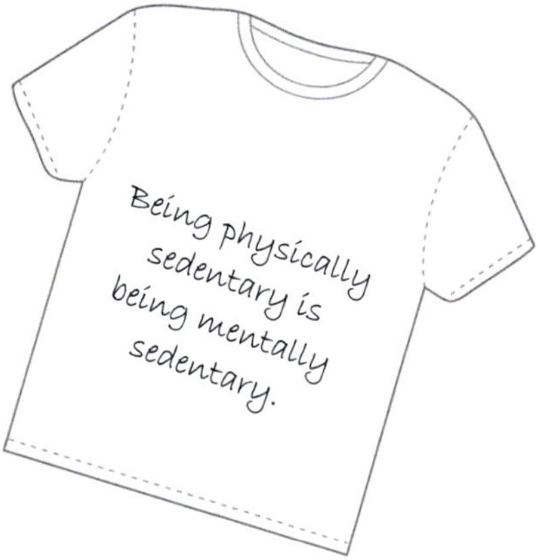

I am grateful; I am sympathetic

I am understanding; I am positive everyday

I am strong; I am dependable

I am honest; I am trustworthy

I will express my gratitude to the universe every day for all that I have and all that I am.

End of Day

A perfect day to spend in the fall sunshine is taking photos and laughing all day.

CONTEMPLATION

I am cared for; I am loved

I am intelligent; I am talented

I am accomplished; I am appreciated

T-Shirt Thought

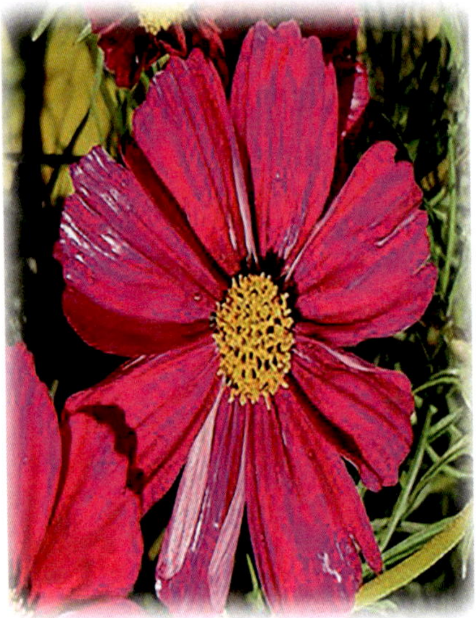

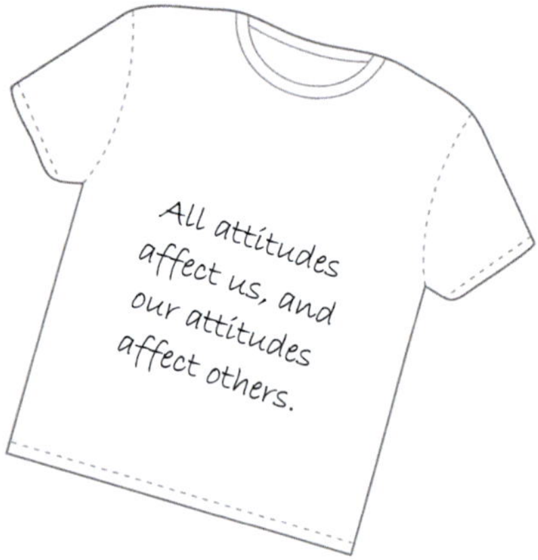

I am grateful; I am sympathetic

I am understanding; I am positive everyday

I am strong; I am dependable

I am honest; I am trustworthy

I will express my gratitude to the universe every day for all that I have and all that I am.

End of Day

It's so easy to make someone happy, just be happy yourself...Smile.

CONTEMPLATION

I am cared for; I am loved

I am intelligent; I am talented

I am accomplished; I am appreciated

T-Shirt Thought

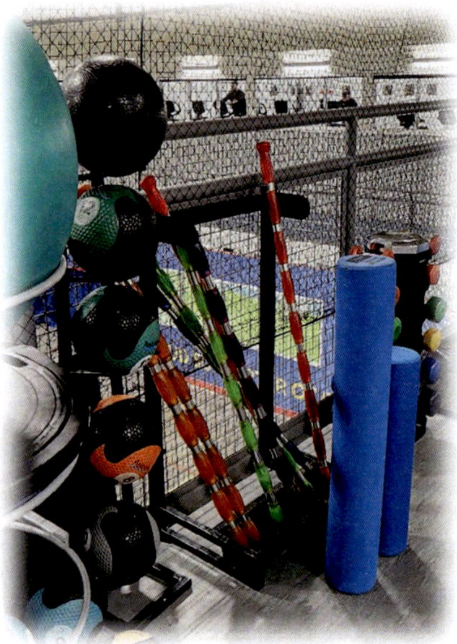

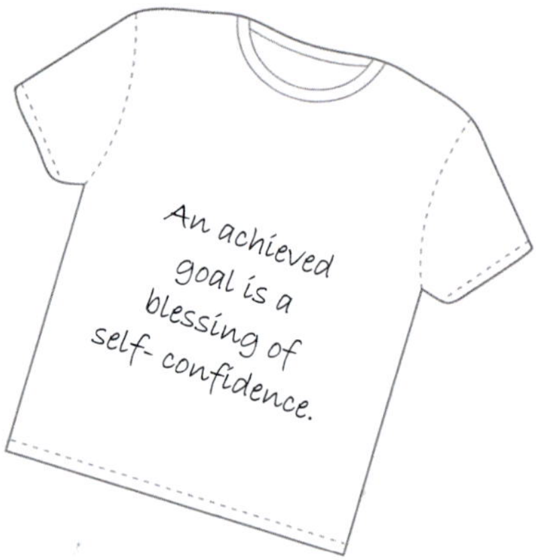

I am grateful; I am sympathetic

I am understanding; I am positive everyday

I am strong; I am dependable

I am honest; I am trustworthy

I will express my gratitude to the universe every day for all that I have and all that I am.

End of Day

Another day, another challenge, another achievement.

CONTEMPLATION

I am cared for; I am loved

I am intelligent; I am talented

I am accomplished; I am appreciated

T-Shirt Thought

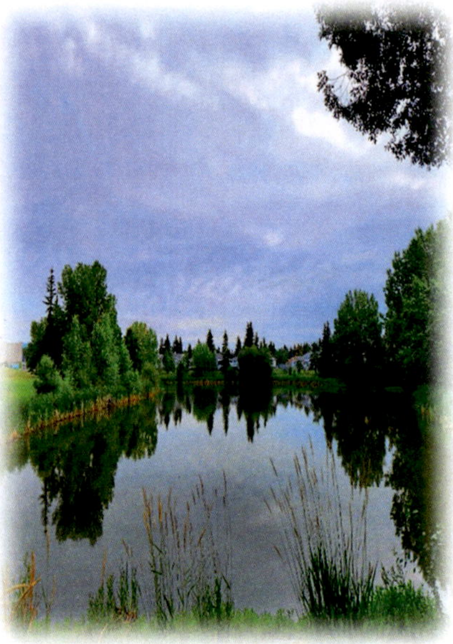

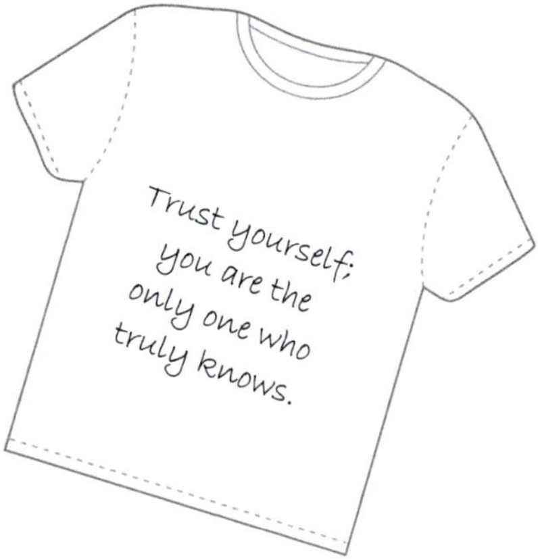

I am grateful; I am sympathetic

I am understanding; I am positive everyday

I am strong; I am dependable

I am honest; I am trustworthy

I will express my gratitude to the universe every day for all that I have and all that I am.

End of Day

Flipping your mindset is not only a success, it's an achievement.

CONTEMPLATION

I am cared for; I am loved

I am intelligent; I am talented

I am accomplished; I am appreciated

T-Shirt Thought

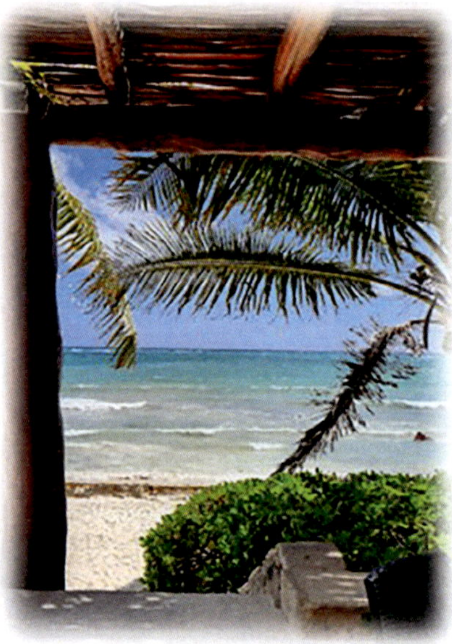

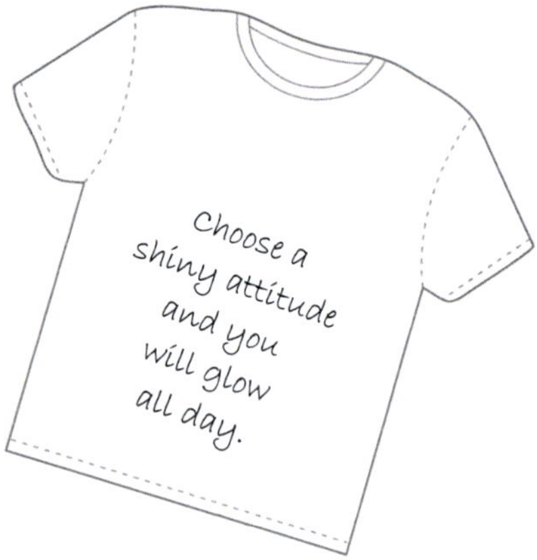

I am grateful; I am sympathetic

I am understanding; I am positive everyday

I am strong; I am dependable

I am honest; I am trustworthy

I will express my gratitude to the universe every day for all that I have and all that I am.

End of Day

Beauty is in the mind, not just the eyes.

CONTEMPLATION

I am cared for; I am loved

I am intelligent; I am talented

I am accomplished; I am appreciated

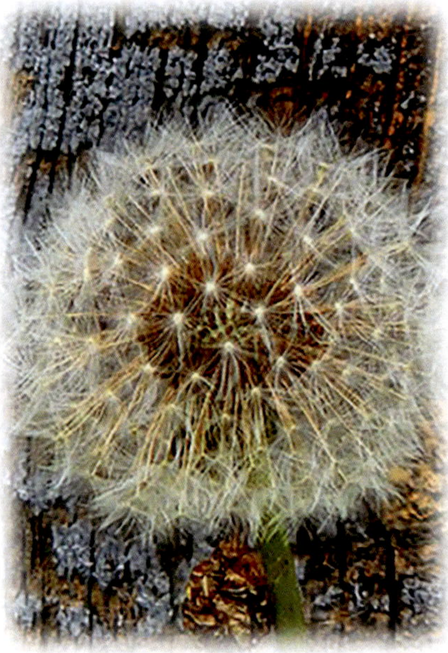

T-Shirt Thought

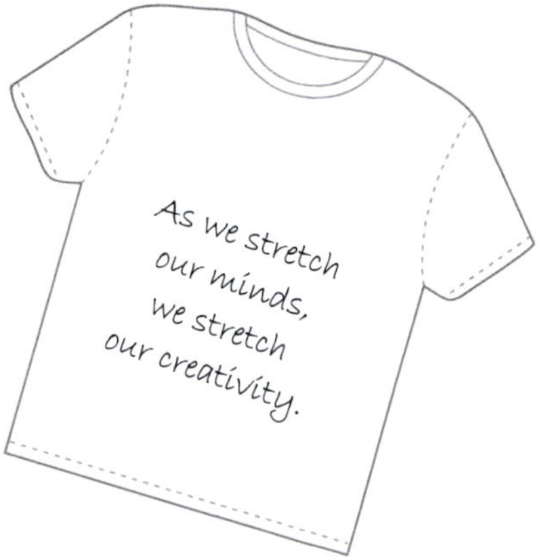

I am grateful; I am sympathetic

I am understanding; I am positive everyday

I am strong; I am dependable

I am honest; I am trustworthy

I will express my gratitude to the universe every day for all that I have and all that I am.

End of Day

The work of a true artist never dies, even when the artist does.

CONTEMPLATION

I am cared for; I am loved

I am intelligent; I am talented

I am accomplished; I am appreciated

T-Shirt Thought

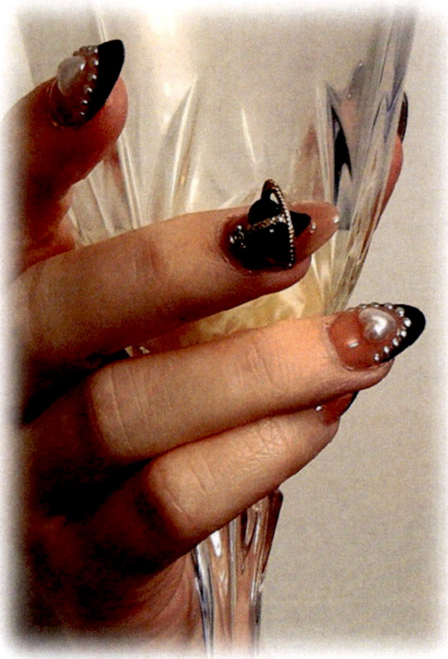

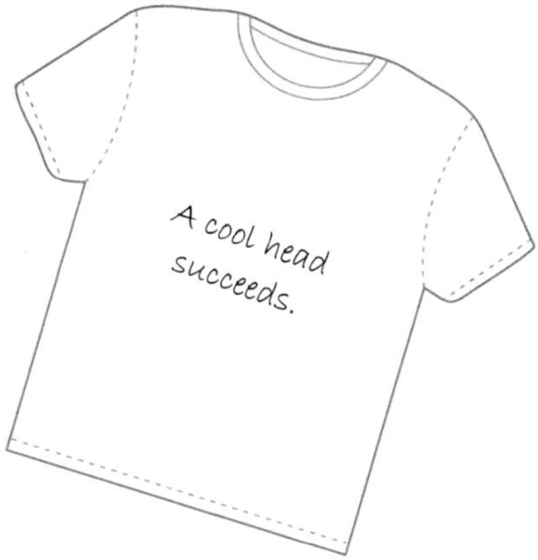

I am grateful; I am sympathetic

I am understanding; I am positive everyday

I am strong; I am dependable

I am honest; I am trustworthy

I will express my gratitude to the universe every day for all that I have and all that I am.

End of Day

Staring down a tough challenge is not only satisfying but uplifting.

CONTEMPLATION

TOGETHER ON THE PATH

I am cared for; I am loved

I am intelligent; I am talented

I am accomplished; I am appreciated

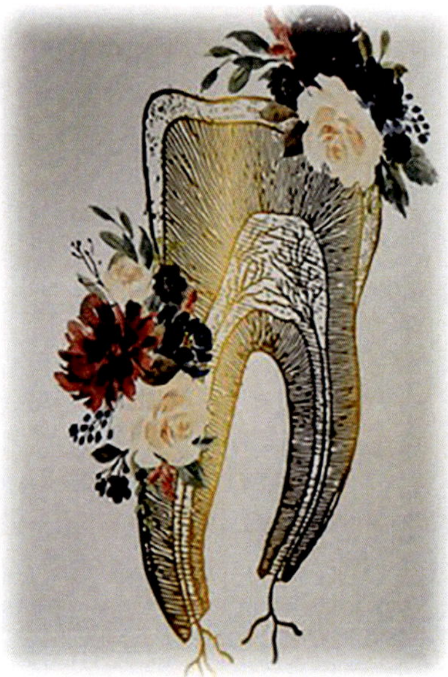

T-Shirt Thought

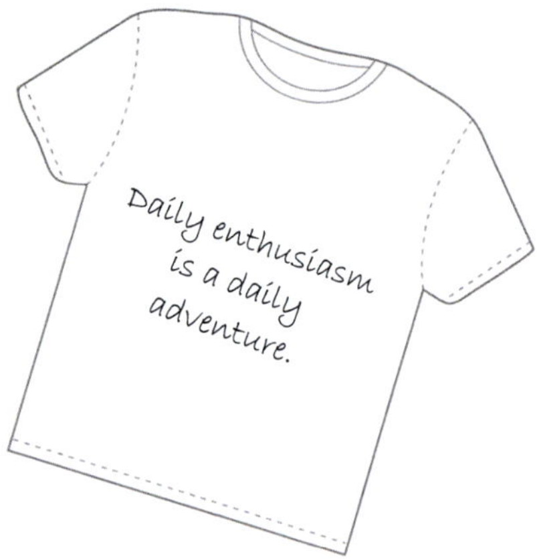

I am grateful; I am sympathetic

I am understanding; I am positive everyday

I am strong; I am dependable

I am honest; I am trustworthy

I will express my gratitude to the universe every day for all that I have and all that I am.

End of Day

Planning to have a good day guarantees a FANTASTIC day.

CONTEMPLATION

I am cared for; I am loved

I am intelligent; I am talented

I am accomplished; I am appreciated

T-Shirt Thought

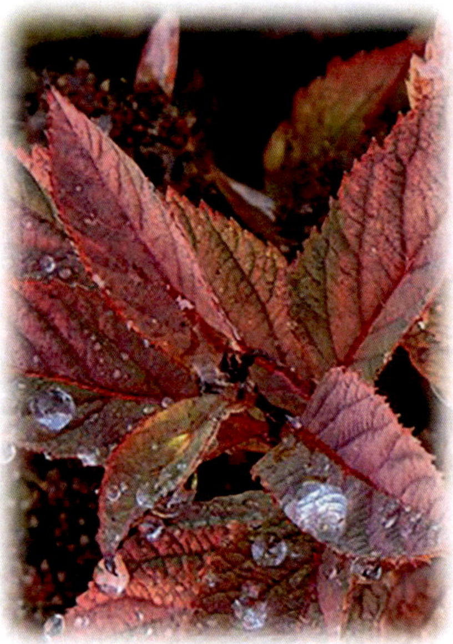

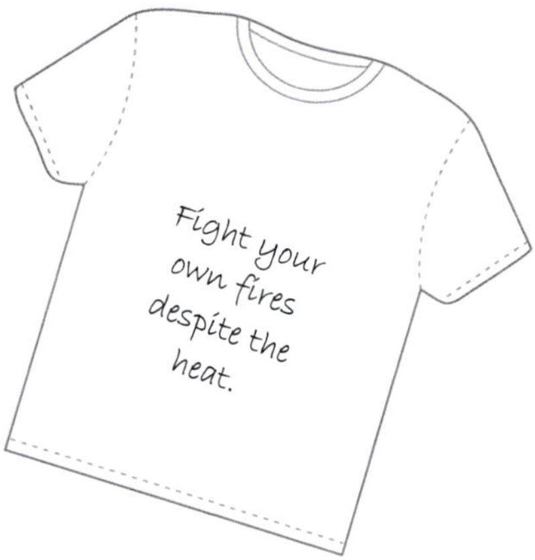

I am grateful; I am sympathetic

I am understanding; I am positive everyday

I am strong; I am dependable

I am honest; I am trustworthy

I will express my gratitude to the universe every day for all that I have and all that I am.

End of Day

Accomplishments are what we do every day.

CONTEMPLATION

TOGETHER ON THE PATH

I am cared for; I am loved

I am intelligent; I am talented

I am accomplished; I am appreciated

T-Shirt Thought

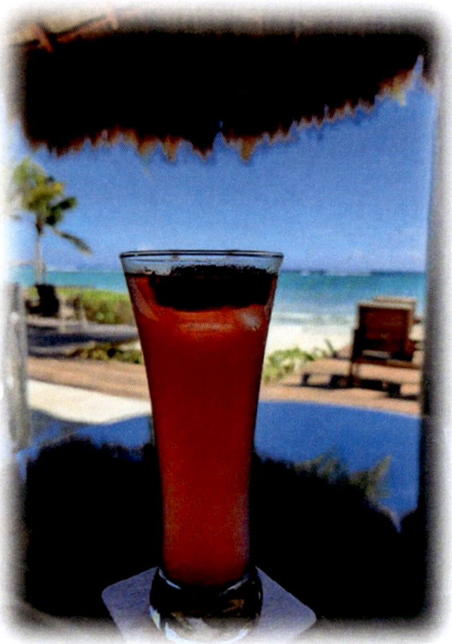

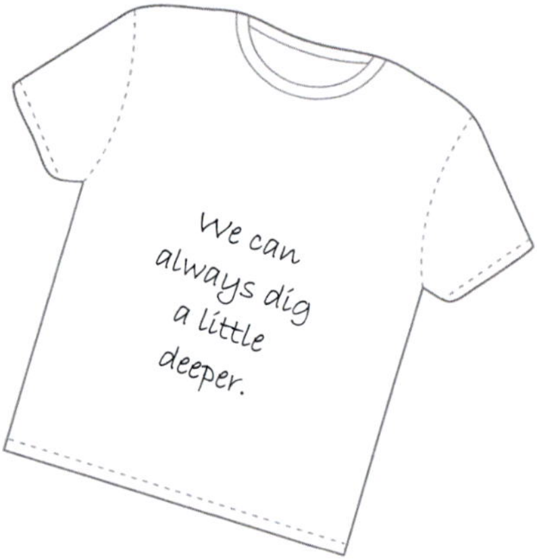

I am grateful; I am sympathetic

I am understanding; I am positive everyday

I am strong; I am dependable

I am honest; I am trustworthy

I will express my gratitude to the universe every day for all that I have and all that I am.

End of Day

We will always amaze ourselves as long as we try.

CONTEMPLATION

I am cared for; I am loved

I am intelligent; I am talented

I am accomplished; I am appreciated

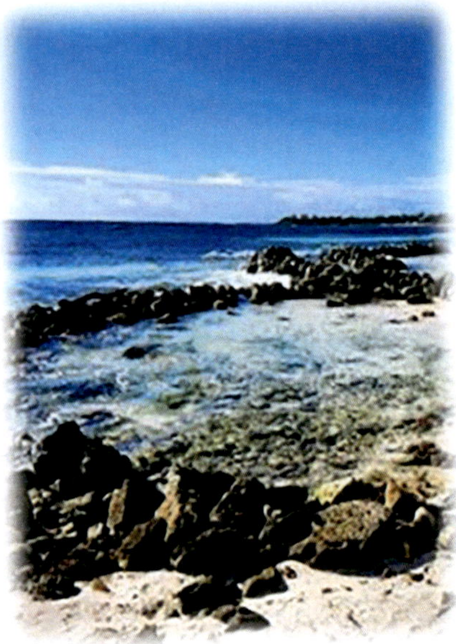

T-Shirt Thought

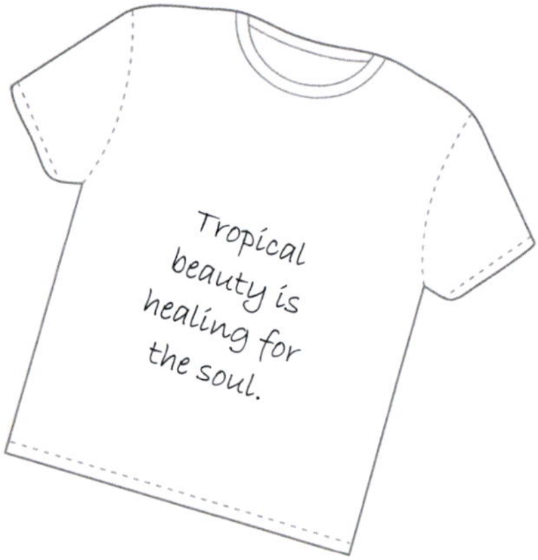

I am grateful; I am sympathetic

I am understanding; I am positive everyday

I am strong; I am dependable

I am honest; I am trustworthy

I will express my gratitude to the universe every day for all that I have and all that I am.

End of Day

If you want good things to happen, relax and let them happen.

CONTEMPLATION

TOGETHER ON THE PATH

I am cared for; I am loved

I am intelligent; I am talented

I am accomplished; I am appreciated

T-Shirt Thought

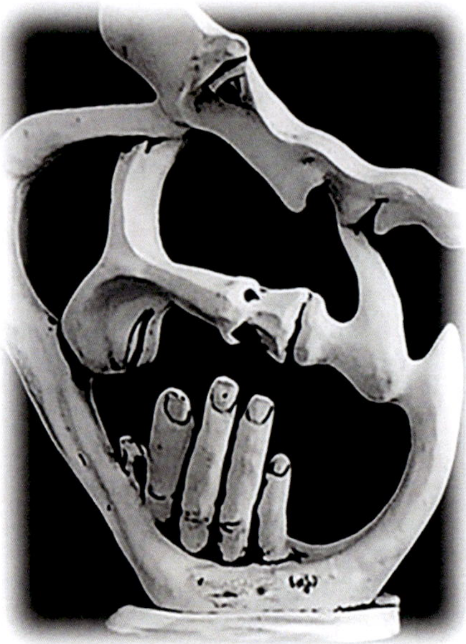

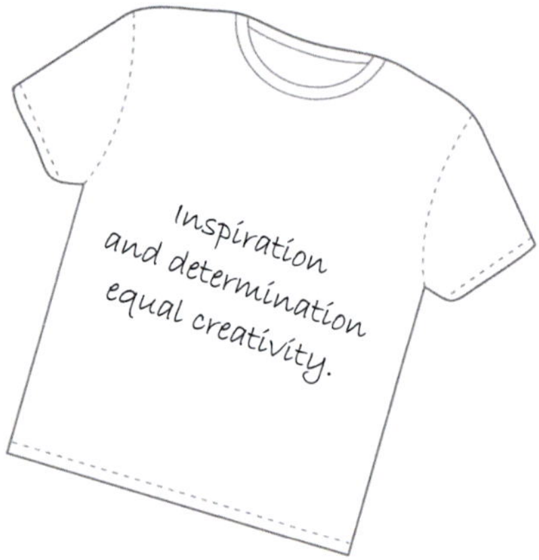

I am grateful; I am sympathetic

I am understanding; I am positive everyday

I am strong; I am dependable

I am honest; I am trustworthy

I will express my gratitude to the universe every day for all that I have and all that I am.

End of Day

Creativity is a daily renewal, an everyday occurrence of beauty and peace.

CONTEMPLATION

I am cared for; I am loved

I am intelligent; I am talented

I am accomplished; I am appreciated

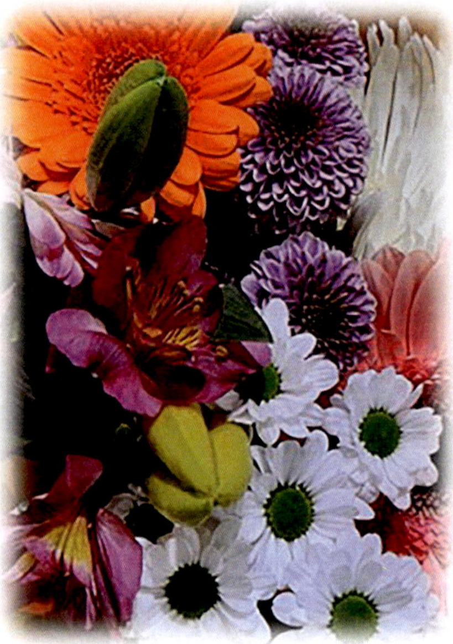

T-Shirt Thought

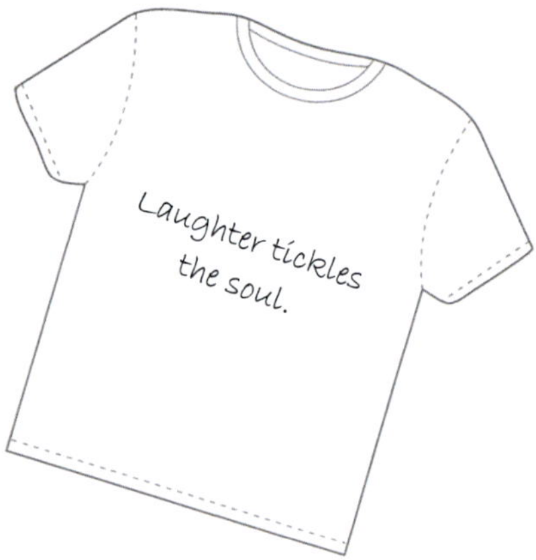

I am grateful; I am sympathetic

I am understanding; I am positive everyday

I am strong; I am dependable

I am honest; I am trustworthy

I will express my gratitude to the universe every day for all that I have and all that I am.

End of Day

A kind word, a smile, and a gesture, will light up the day every time.

CONTEMPLATION

I am cared for; I am loved

I am intelligent; I am talented

I am accomplished; I am appreciated

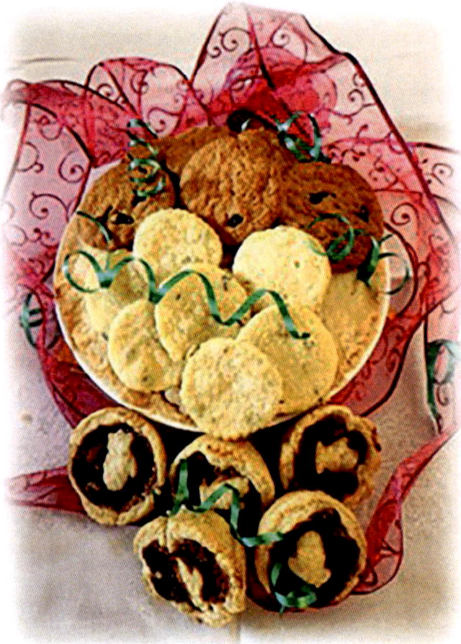

T-Shirt Thought

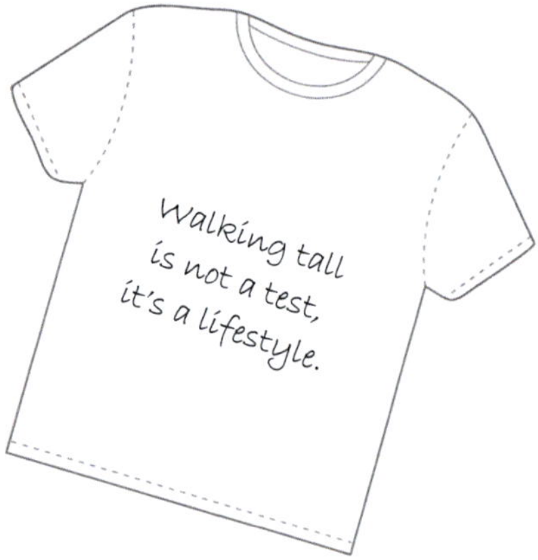

I am grateful; I am sympathetic

I am understanding; I am positive everyday

I am strong; I am dependable

I am honest; I am trustworthy

I will express my gratitude to the universe every day for all that I have and all that I am.

End of Day

An overwhelming day does not have to be a negative day. It can be energizing and exciting.

CONTEMPLATION

I am cared for; I am loved

I am intelligent; I am talented

I am accomplished; I am appreciated

T-Shirt Thought

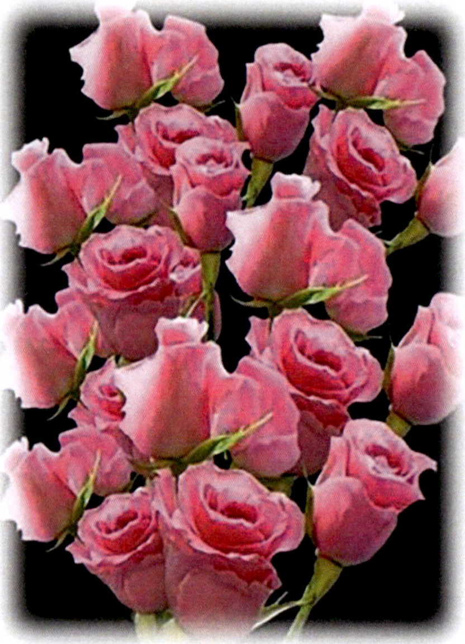

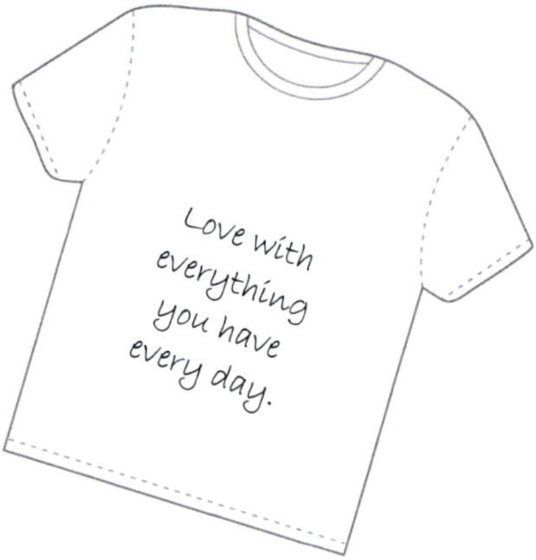

I am grateful; I am sympathetic

I am understanding; I am positive everyday

I am strong; I am dependable

I am honest; I am trustworthy

I will express my gratitude to the universe every day for all that I have and all that I am.

End of Day

When two people that I love meet for the first time, my heart sings.

CONTEMPLATION

I am cared for; I am loved

I am intelligent; I am talented

I am accomplished; I am appreciated

T-Shirt Thought

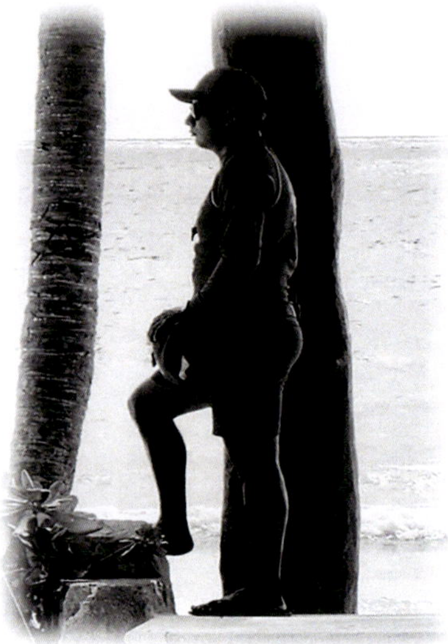

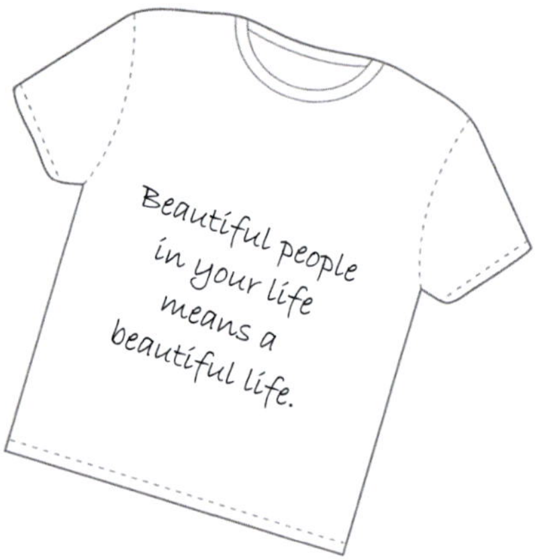

I am grateful; I am sympathetic

I am understanding; I am positive everyday

I am strong; I am dependable

I am honest; I am trustworthy

I will express my gratitude to the universe every day for all that I have and all that I am.

End of Day

Laughter with a stranger has the potential to become laughter with a friend.

CONTEMPLATION

I am cared for; I am loved

I am intelligent; I am talented

I am accomplished; I am appreciated

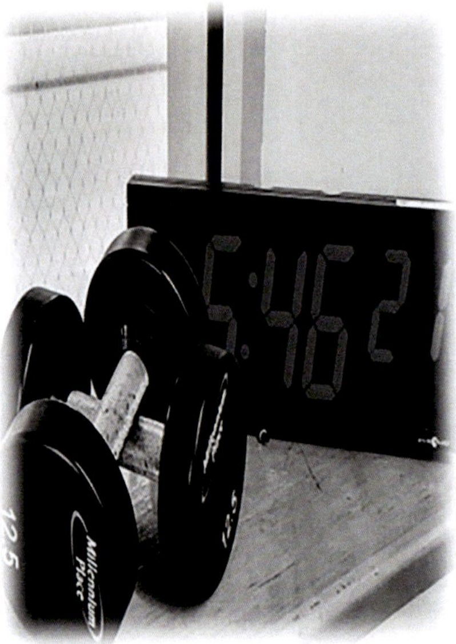

T-Shirt Thought

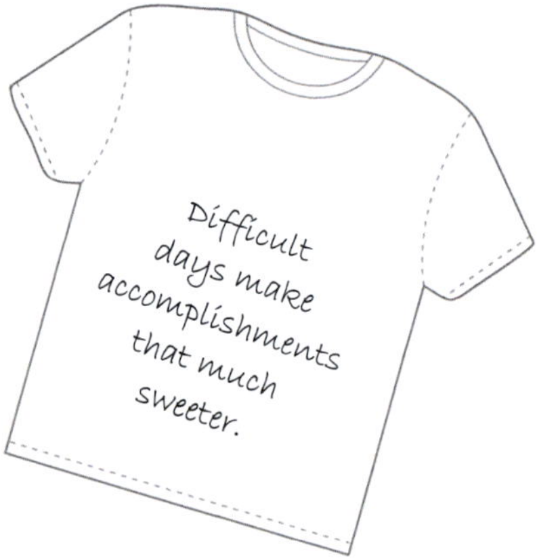

I am grateful; I am sympathetic

I am understanding; I am positive everyday

I am strong; I am dependable

I am honest; I am trustworthy

I will express my gratitude to the universe every day for all that I have and all that I am.

End of Day

If we don't overthink a situation, the situation becomes less difficult to manage and change.

CONTEMPLATION

I am cared for; I am loved

I am intelligent; I am talented

I am accomplished; I am appreciated

T-Shirt Thought

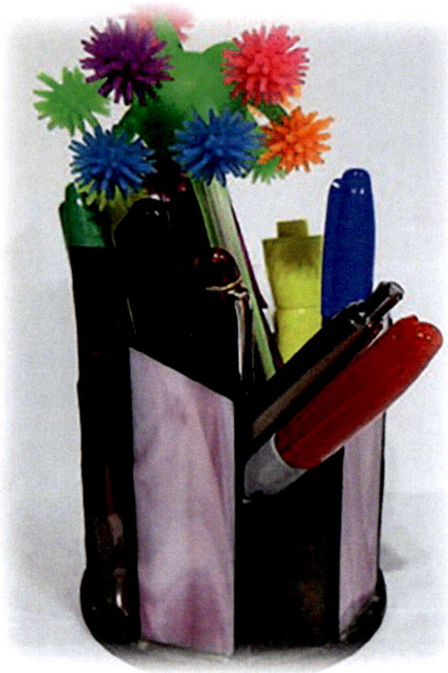

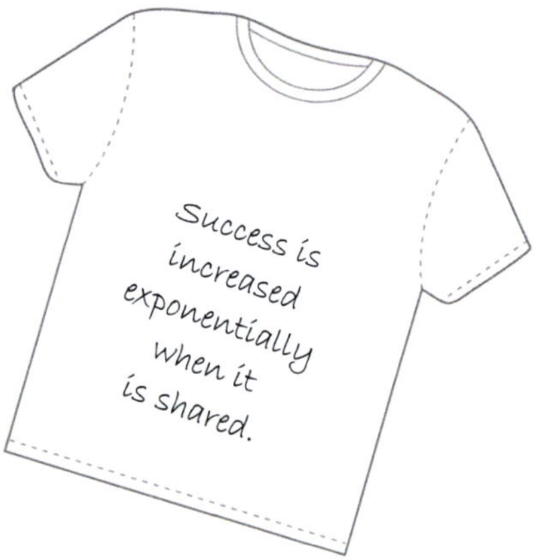

I am grateful; I am sympathetic

I am understanding; I am positive everyday

I am strong; I am dependable

I am honest; I am trustworthy

I will express my gratitude to the universe every day for all that I have and all that I am.

End of Day

Patience and a cool head mean success without stress.

CONTEMPLATION

I am cared for; I am loved

I am intelligent; I am talented

I am accomplished; I am appreciated

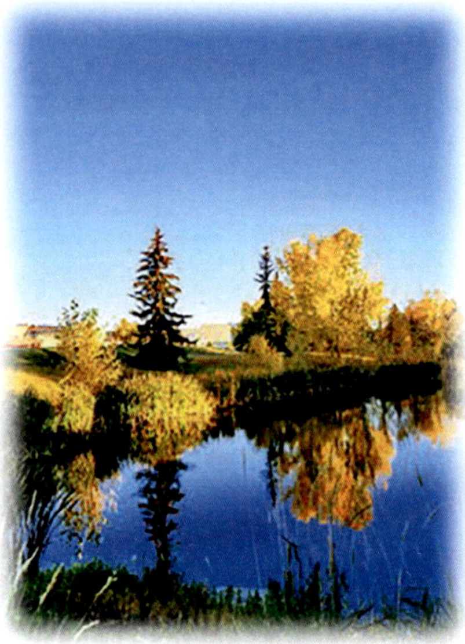

T-Shirt Thought

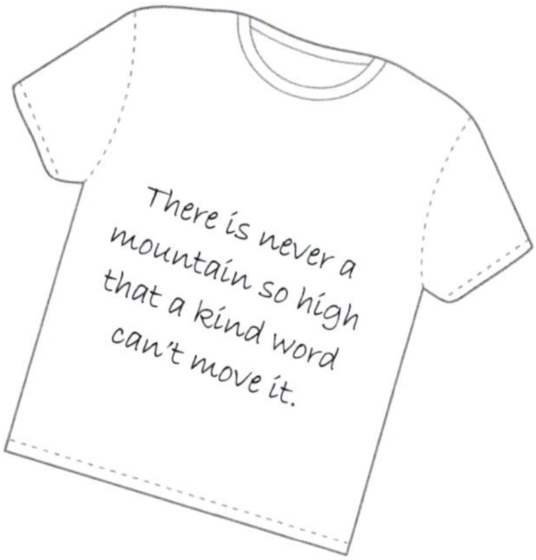

I am grateful; I am sympathetic

I am understanding; I am positive everyday

I am strong; I am dependable

I am honest; I am trustworthy

I will express my gratitude to the universe every day for all that I have and all that I am.

End of Day

Not every day will be perfect, but every day has the potential.

CONTEMPLATION

I am cared for; I am loved

I am intelligent; I am talented

I am accomplished; I am appreciated

T-Shirt Thought

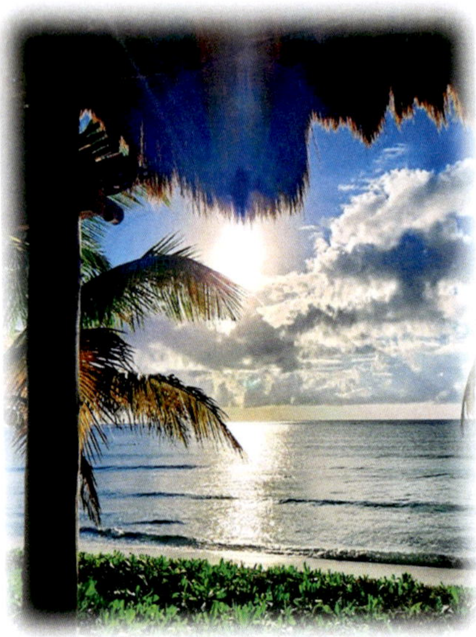

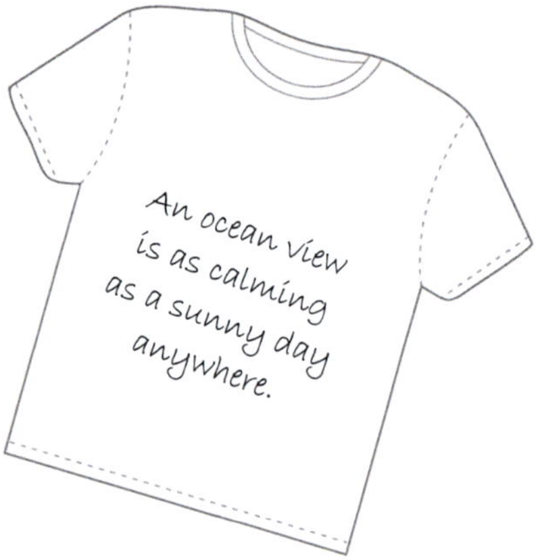

I am grateful; I am sympathetic

I am understanding; I am positive everyday

I am strong; I am dependable

I am honest; I am trustworthy

I will express my gratitude to the universe every day for all that I have and all that I am.

End of Day

When you feel gratitude, you truly are at peace.

CONTEMPLATION

TOGETHER ON THE PATH

I am cared for; I am loved

I am intelligent; I am talented

I am accomplished; I am appreciated

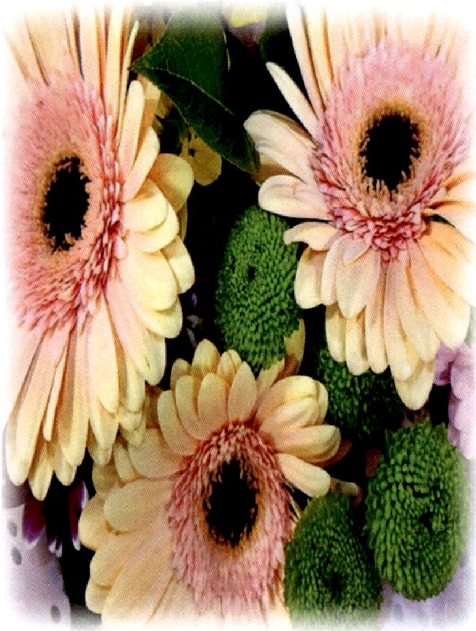

T-Shirt Thought

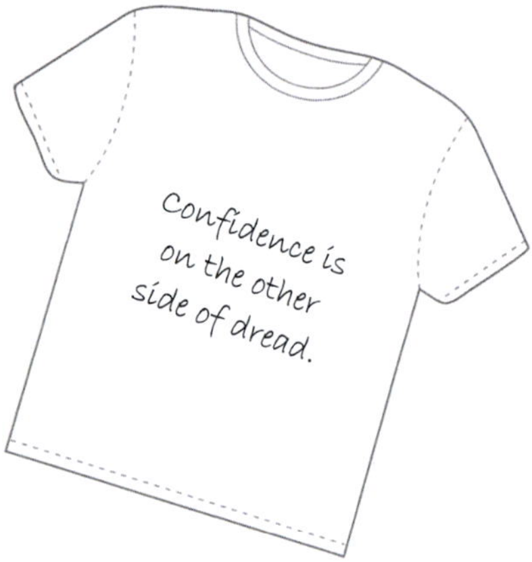

I am grateful; I am sympathetic

I am understanding; I am positive everyday

I am strong; I am dependable

I am honest; I am trustworthy

I will express my gratitude to the universe every day for all that I have and all that I am.

End of Day

The effort made to change a negative day to a positive one pays off exponentially.

CONTEMPLATION

I am cared for; I am loved

I am intelligent; I am talented

I am accomplished; I am appreciated

T-Shirt Thought

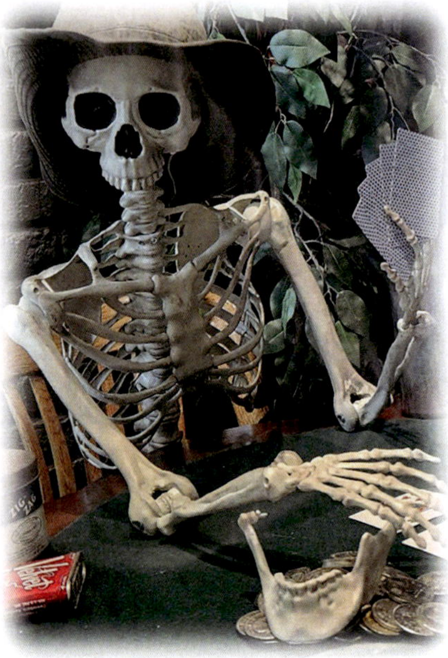

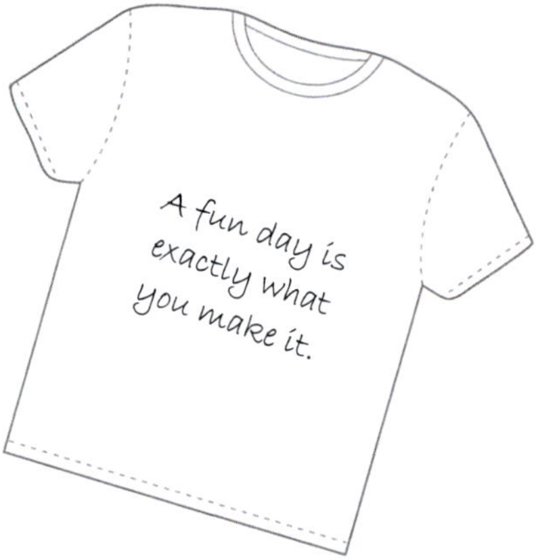

I am grateful; I am sympathetic

I am understanding; I am positive everyday

I am strong; I am dependable

I am honest; I am trustworthy

I will express my gratitude to the universe every day for all that I have and all that I am.

End of Day

A multitask day is a fun day.

CONTEMPLATION

I am cared for; I am loved

I am intelligent; I am talented

I am accomplished; I am appreciated

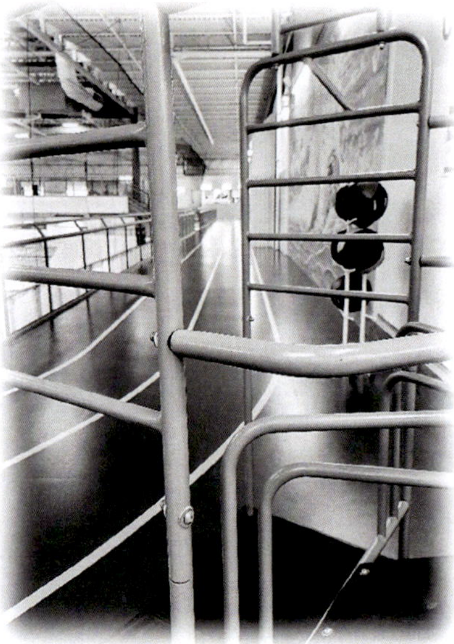

T-Shirt Thought

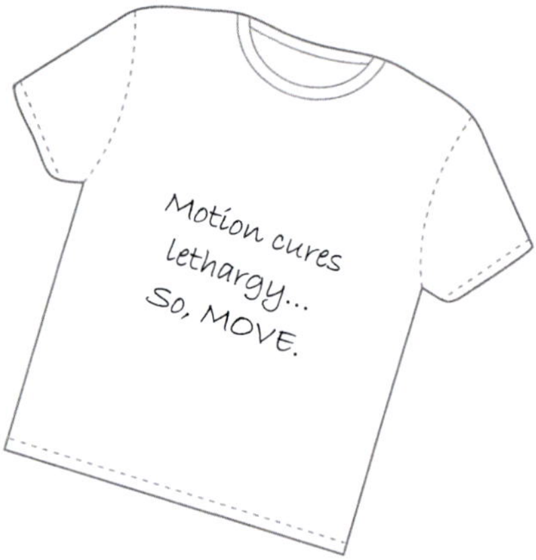

I am grateful; I am sympathetic

I am understanding; I am positive everyday

I am strong; I am dependable

I am honest; I am trustworthy

I will express my gratitude to the universe every day for all that I have and all that I am.

End of Day

When you power through exhaustion, you power up your day.

CONTEMPLATION

I am cared for; I am loved

I am intelligent; I am talented

I am accomplished; I am appreciated

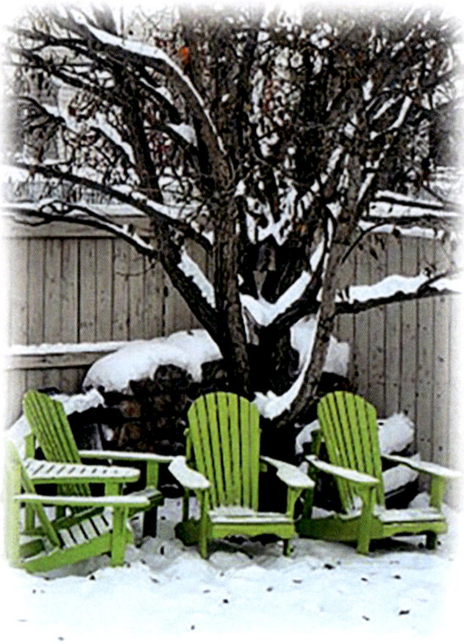

T-Shirt Thought

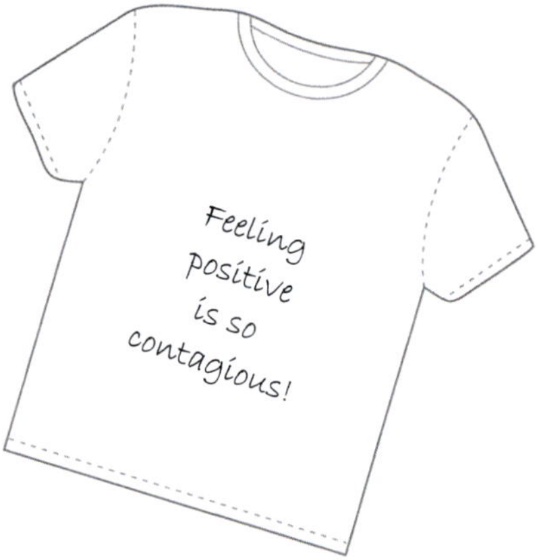

I am grateful; I am sympathetic

I am understanding; I am positive everyday

I am strong; I am dependable

I am honest; I am trustworthy

I will express my gratitude to the universe every day for all that I have and all that I am.

End of Day

Pain shared with a loved one quickly turns to delight.

CONTEMPLATION

I am cared for; I am loved

I am intelligent; I am talented

I am accomplished; I am appreciated

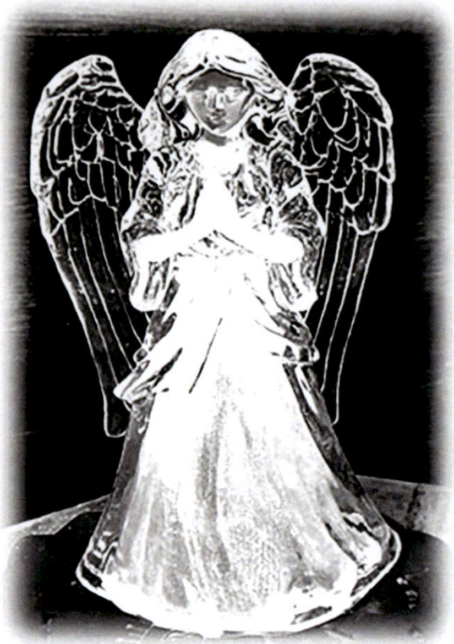

T-Shirt Thought

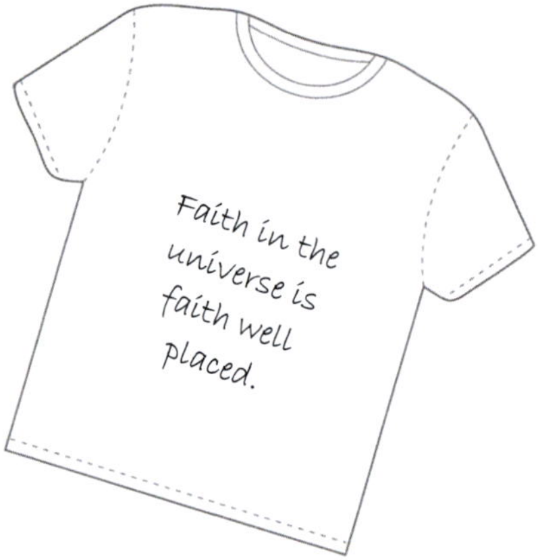

I am grateful; I am sympathetic

I am understanding; I am positive everyday

I am strong; I am dependable

I am honest; I am trustworthy

I will express my gratitude to the universe every day for all that I have and all that I am.

End of Day

The touch of a summer breeze is like an angel's kiss.

CONTEMPLATION

I am cared for; I am loved

I am intelligent; I am talented

I am accomplished; I am appreciated

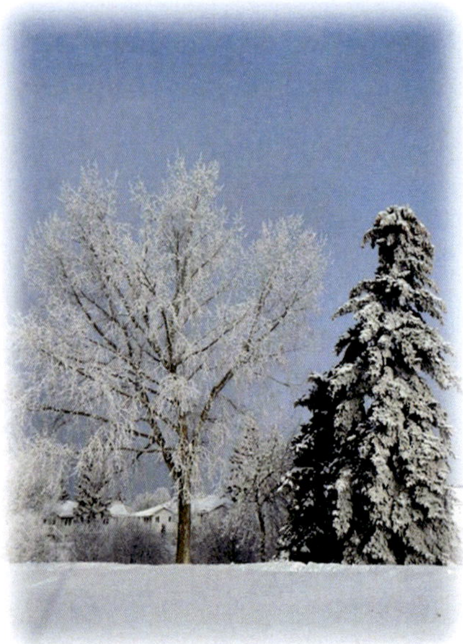

T-Shirt Thought

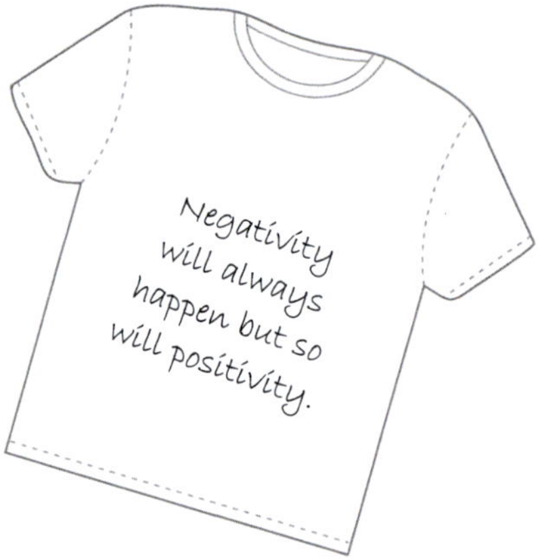

I am grateful; I am sympathetic

I am understanding; I am positive everyday

I am strong; I am dependable

I am honest; I am trustworthy

I will express my gratitude to the universe every day for all that I have and all that I am.

End of Day

When something feels negative, stare it down and make it positive.

CONTEMPLATION

I am cared for; I am loved

I am intelligent; I am talented

I am accomplished; I am appreciated

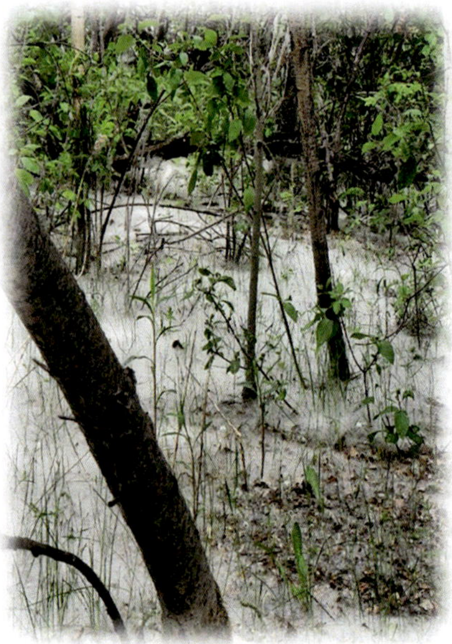

T-Shirt Thought

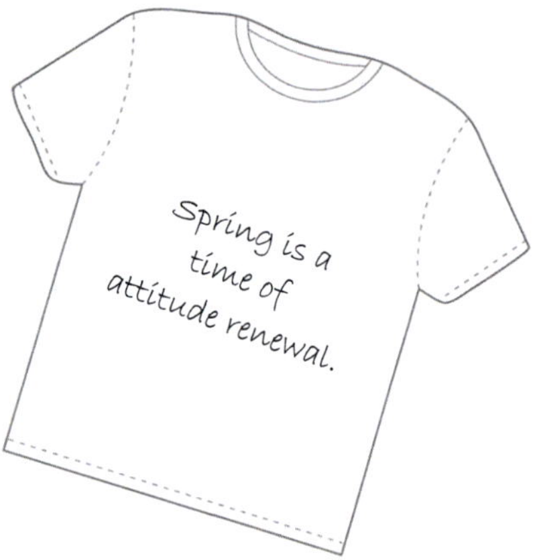

I am grateful; I am sympathetic

I am understanding; I am positive everyday

I am strong; I am dependable

I am honest; I am trustworthy

I will express my gratitude to the universe every day for all that I have and all that I am.

End of Day

Spring really is a time of renewal, love, energy, creativity, and mostly, attitude.

CONTEMPLATION

I am cared for; I am loved

I am intelligent; I am talented

I am accomplished; I am appreciated

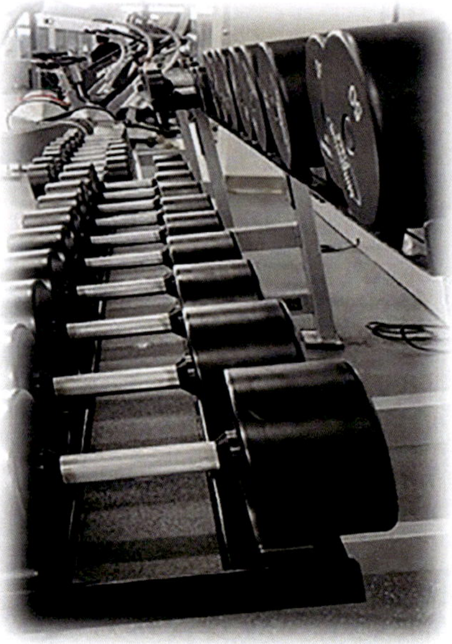

T-Shirt Thought

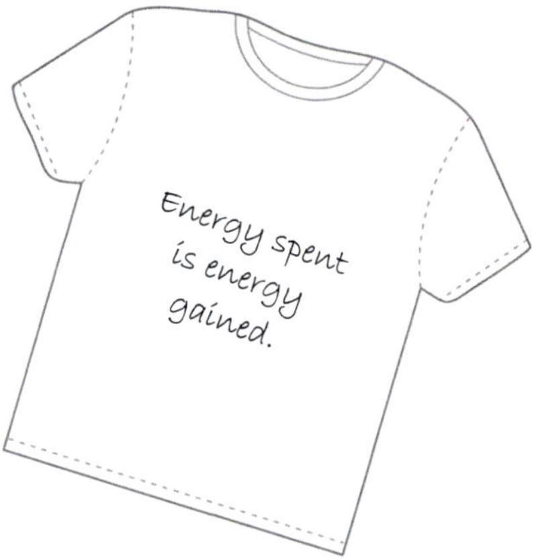

I am grateful; I am sympathetic

I am understanding; I am positive everyday

I am strong; I am dependable

I am honest; I am trustworthy

I will express my gratitude to the universe every day for all that I have and all that I am.

End of Day

Knowing we have things to do is not overwhelming, it is energizing.

CONTEMPLATION

I am cared for; I am loved

I am intelligent; I am talented

I am accomplished; I am appreciated

T-Shirt Thought

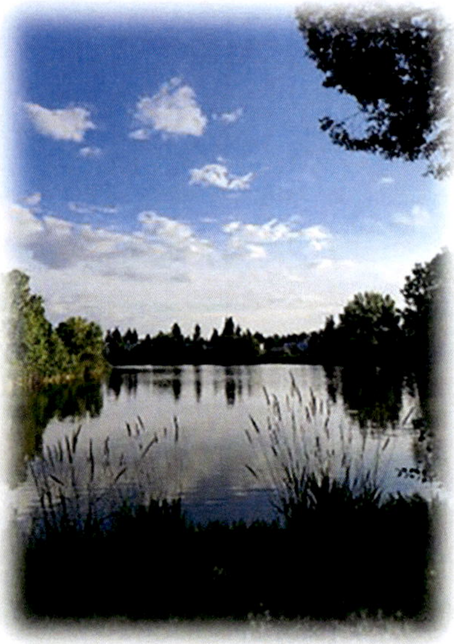

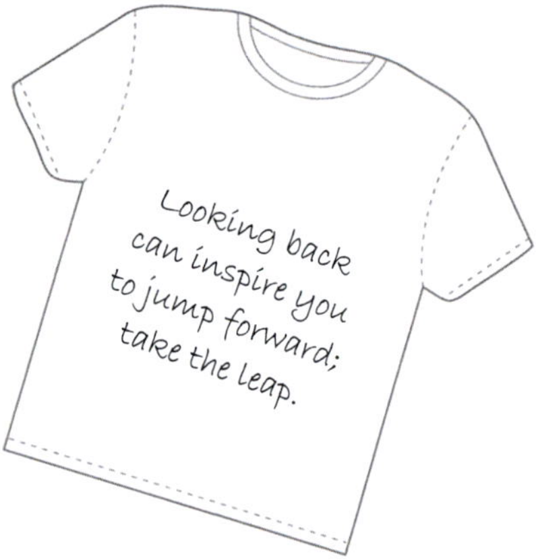

I am grateful; I am sympathetic

I am understanding; I am positive everyday

I am strong; I am dependable

I am honest; I am trustworthy

I will express my gratitude to the universe every day for all that I have and all that I am.

End of Day

Don't stop and think about it, just take a leap and DO IT.

CONTEMPLATION

I am cared for; I am loved

I am intelligent; I am talented

I am accomplished; I am appreciated

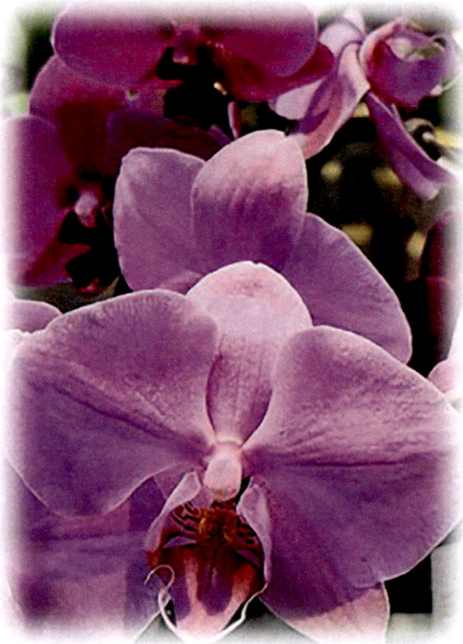

T-Shirt Thought

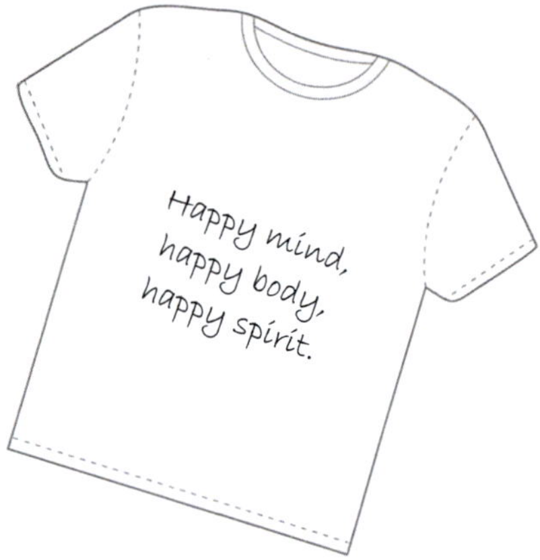

I am grateful; I am sympathetic

I am understanding; I am positive everyday

I am strong; I am dependable

I am honest; I am trustworthy

I will express my gratitude to the universe every day for all that I have and all that I am.

End of Day

Whenever your mind rules your body, your body becomes happy.

CONTEMPLATION

I am cared for; I am loved

I am intelligent; I am talented

I am accomplished; I am appreciated

T-Shirt Thought

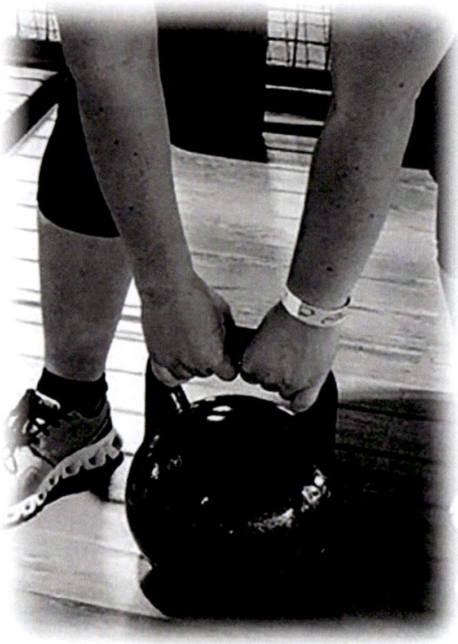

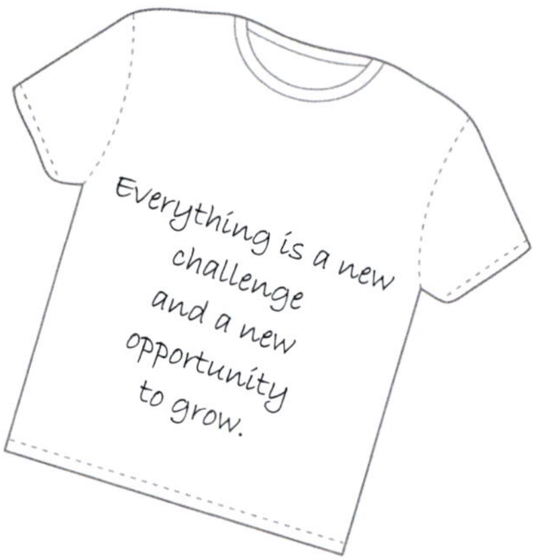

I am grateful; I am sympathetic

I am understanding; I am positive everyday

I am strong; I am dependable

I am honest; I am trustworthy

I will express my gratitude to the universe every day for all that I have and all that I am.

End of Day

Highs and lows are part of every day. Personal strength is dealing with them.

CONTEMPLATION

I am cared for; I am loved

I am intelligent; I am talented

I am accomplished; I am appreciated

T-Shirt Thought

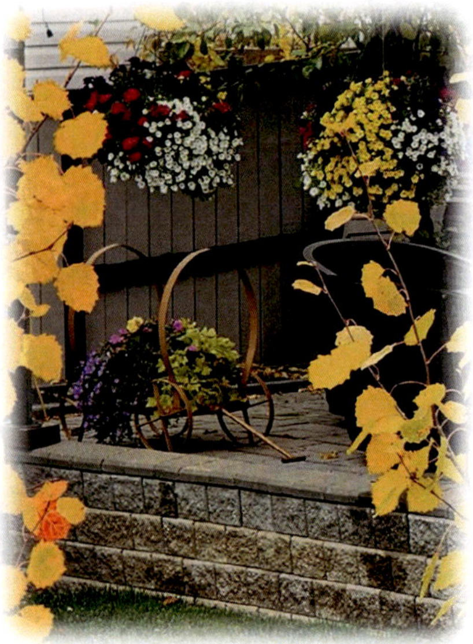

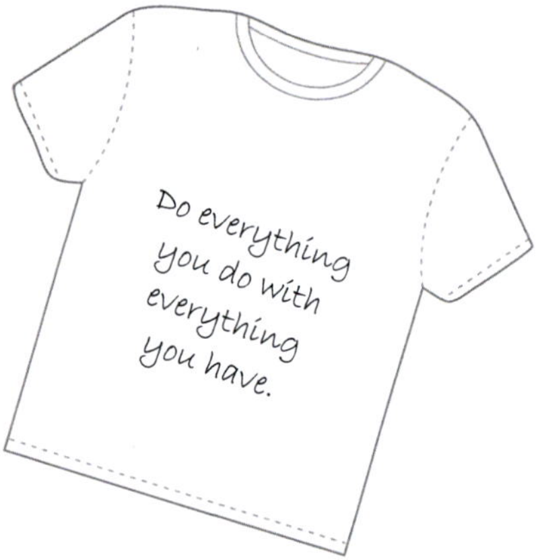

I am grateful; I am sympathetic

I am understanding; I am positive everyday

I am strong; I am dependable

I am honest; I am trustworthy

I will express my gratitude to the universe every day for all that I have and all that I am.

End of Day

There is a sense of satisfaction in knowing you have done all you can.

CONTEMPLATION

I am cared for; I am loved

I am intelligent; I am talented

I am accomplished; I am appreciated

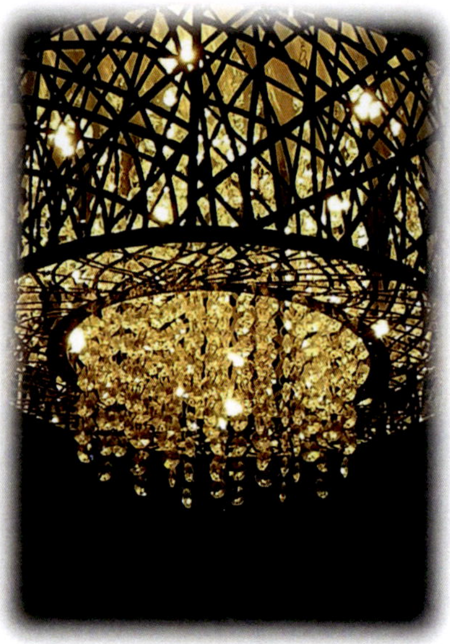

T-Shirt Thought

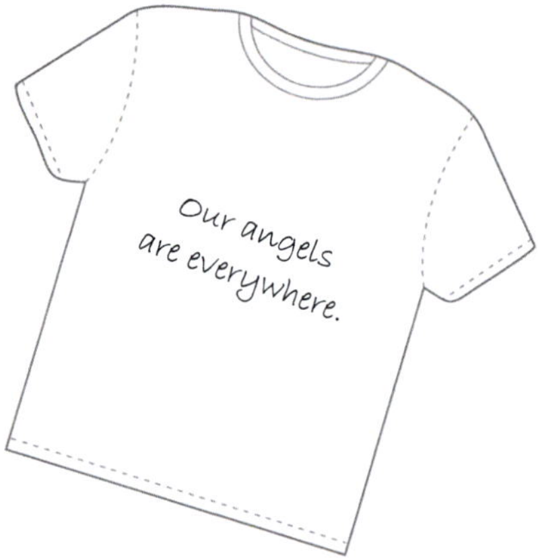

I am grateful; I am sympathetic

I am understanding; I am positive everyday

I am strong; I am dependable

I am honest; I am trustworthy

I will express my gratitude to the universe every day for all that I have and all that I am.

End of Day

The universe is watching. All we need to do is acknowledge it.

CONTEMPLATION

TOGETHER ON THE PATH

I am cared for; I am loved

I am intelligent; I am talented

I am accomplished; I am appreciated

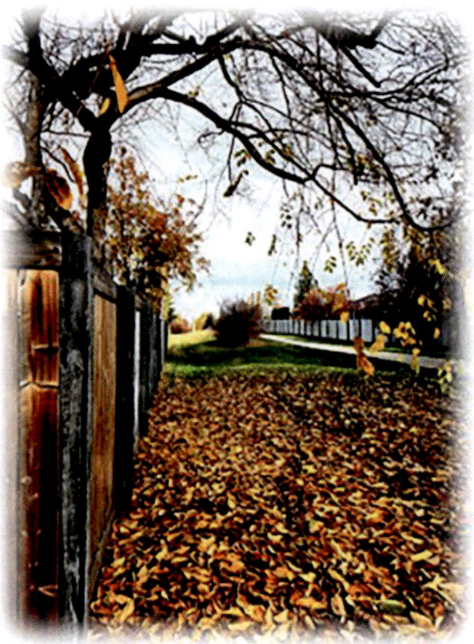

T-Shirt Thought

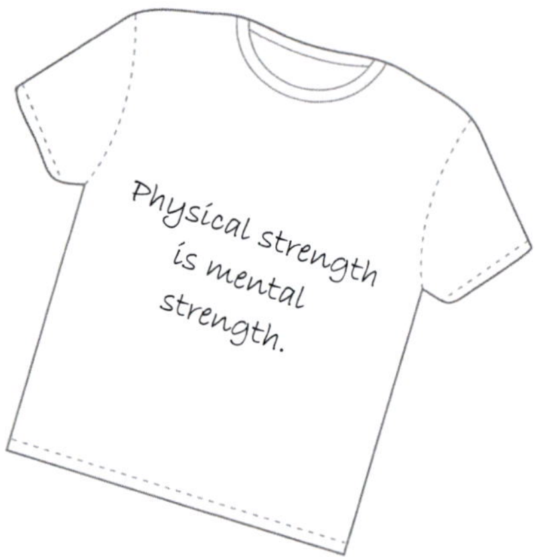

I am grateful; I am sympathetic

I am understanding; I am positive everyday

I am strong; I am dependable

I am honest; I am trustworthy

I will express my gratitude to the universe every day for all that I have and all that I am.

End of Day

Mental health promotes physical healing.

CONTEMPLATION

I am cared for; I am loved

I am intelligent; I am talented

I am accomplished; I am appreciated

T-Shirt Thought

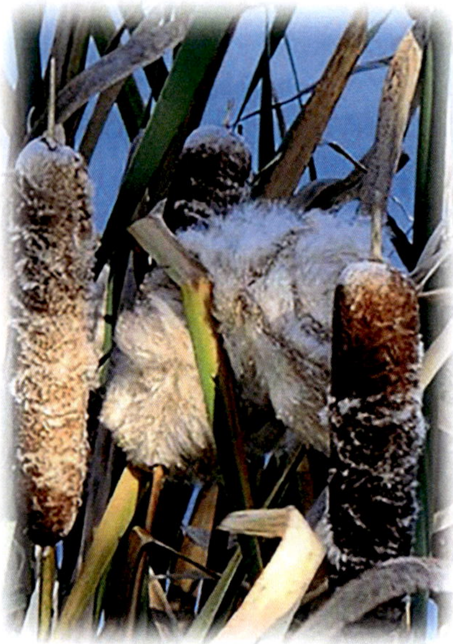

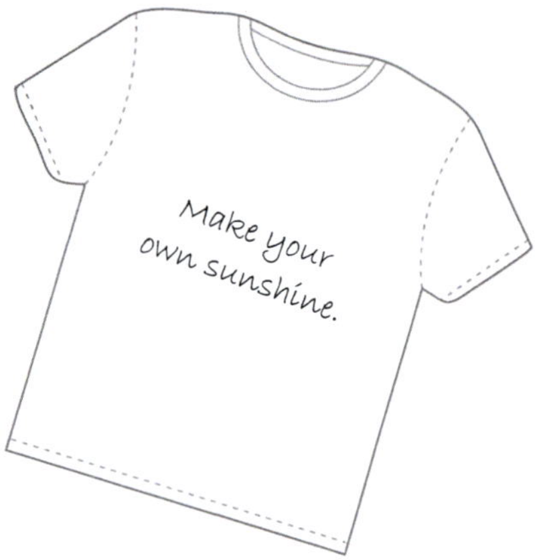

I am grateful; I am sympathetic

I am understanding; I am positive everyday

I am strong; I am dependable

I am honest; I am trustworthy

I will express my gratitude to the universe every day for all that I have and all that I am.

End of Day

Doing something you just don't feel like doing is twice as satisfying.

CONTEMPLATION

I am cared for; I am loved

I am intelligent; I am talented

I am accomplished; I am appreciated

T-Shirt Thought

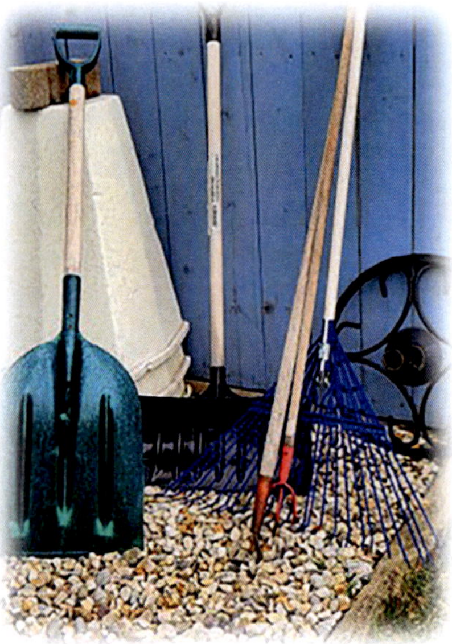

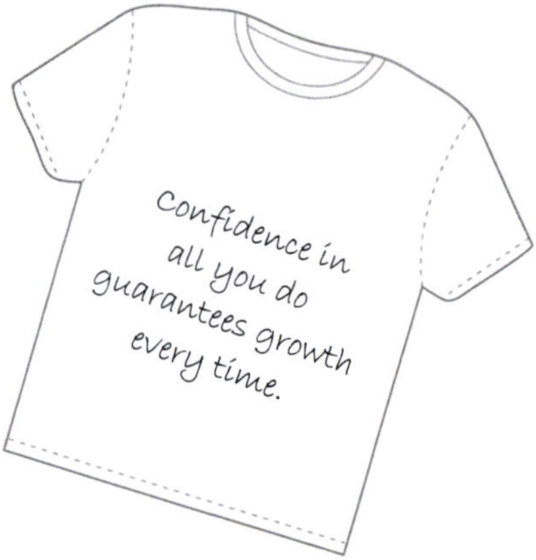

I am grateful; I am sympathetic

I am understanding; I am positive everyday

I am strong; I am dependable

I am honest; I am trustworthy

I will express my gratitude to the universe every day for all that I have and all that I am.

End of Day

Every successful struggle increases our confidence.

CONTEMPLATION

TOGETHER ON THE PATH

I am cared for; I am loved

I am intelligent; I am talented

I am accomplished; I am appreciated

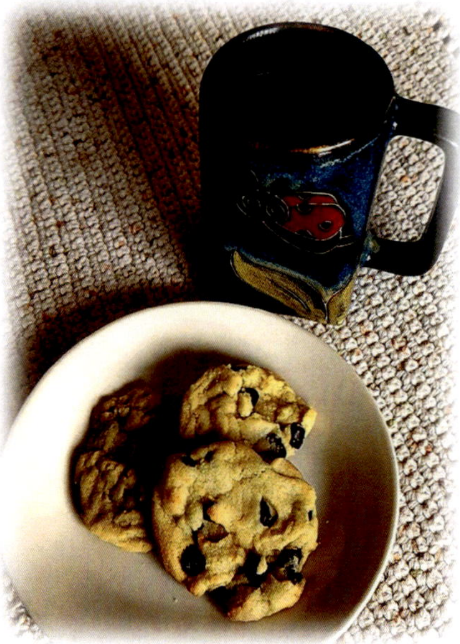

T-Shirt Thought

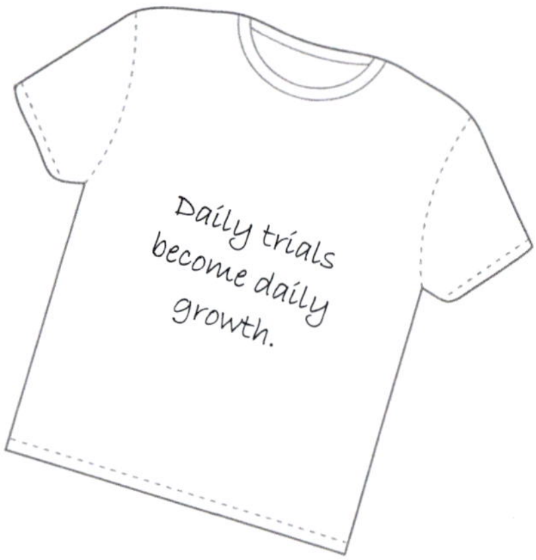

I am grateful; I am sympathetic

I am understanding; I am positive everyday

I am strong; I am dependable

I am honest; I am trustworthy

I will express my gratitude to the universe every day for all that I have and all that I am.

End of Day

Chaos and confusion need not overwhelm you. A minute at a time will get you through it.

CONTEMPLATION

TOGETHER ON THE PATH

I am cared for; I am loved

I am intelligent; I am talented

I am accomplished; I am appreciated

T-Shirt Thought

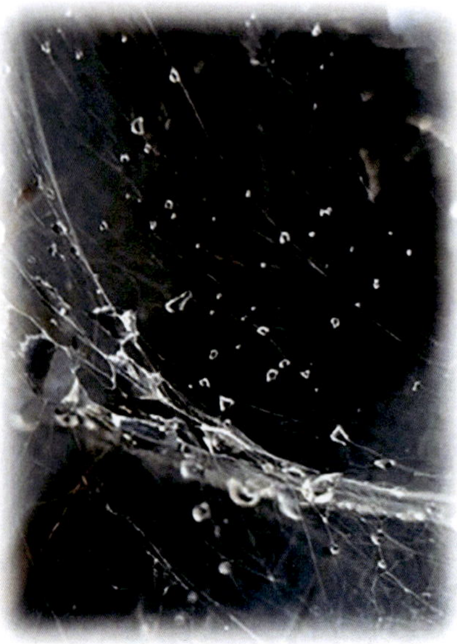

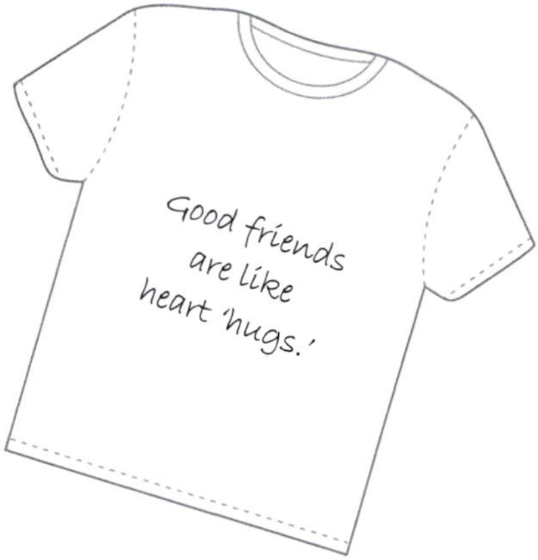

I am grateful; I am sympathetic

I am understanding; I am positive everyday

I am strong; I am dependable

I am honest; I am trustworthy

I will express my gratitude to the universe every day for all that I have and all that I am.

End of Day

Reconnecting with old friends is an absolute privilege.

CONTEMPLATION

TOGETHER ON THE PATH

I am cared for; I am loved

I am intelligent; I am talented

I am accomplished; I am appreciated

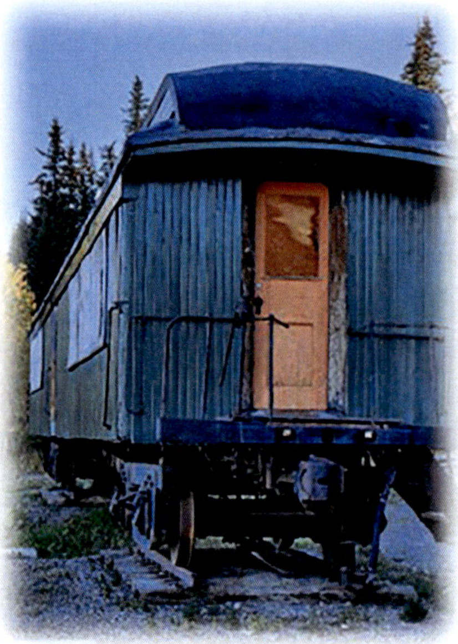

T-Shirt Thought

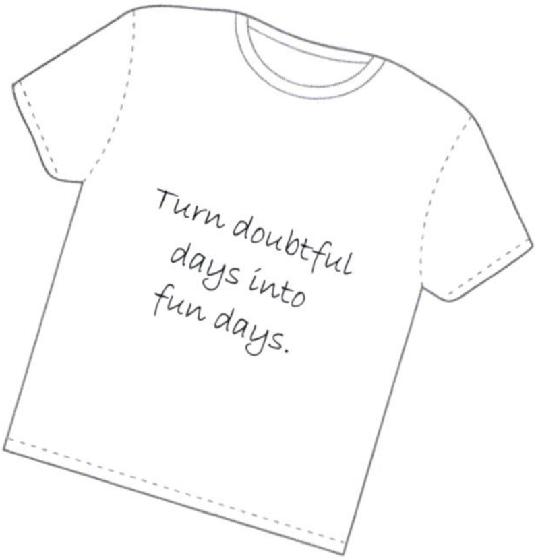

I am grateful; I am sympathetic

I am understanding; I am positive everyday

I am strong; I am dependable

I am honest; I am trustworthy

I will express my gratitude to the universe every day for all that I have and all that I am.

End of Day

Do good things happen because of a good mindset or does a good mindset bring on good things?

CONTEMPLATION

TOGETHER ON THE PATH

I am cared for; I am loved

I am intelligent; I am talented

I am accomplished; I am appreciated

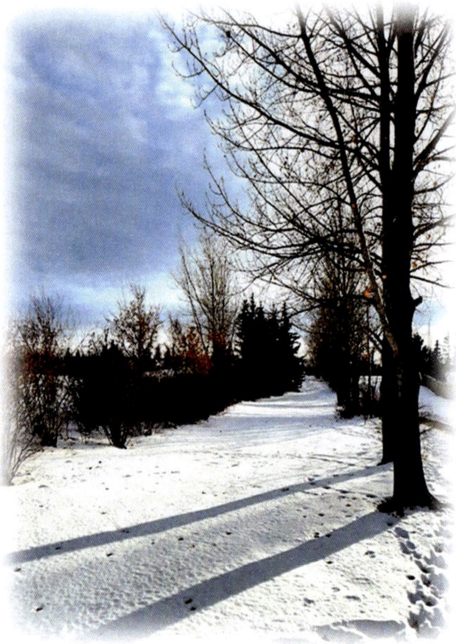

T-Shirt Thought

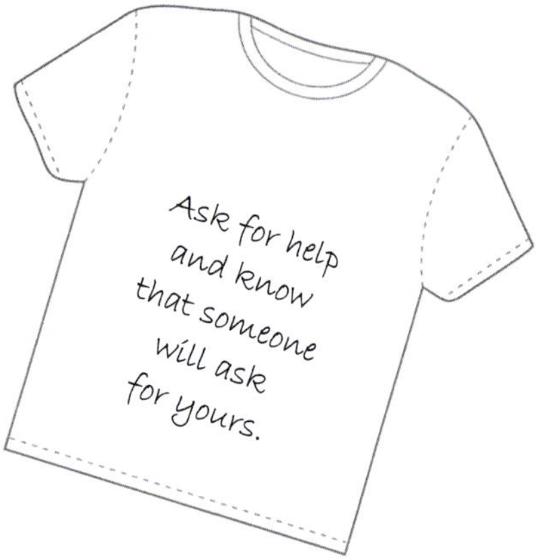

I am grateful; I am sympathetic

I am understanding; I am positive everyday

I am strong; I am dependable

I am honest; I am trustworthy

I will express my gratitude to the universe every day for all that I have and all that I am.

End of Day

Baring the soul is opening the heart…peaceful, vulnerable, content.

CONTEMPLATION

TOGETHER ON THE PATH

I am cared for; I am loved

I am intelligent; I am talented

I am accomplished; I am appreciated

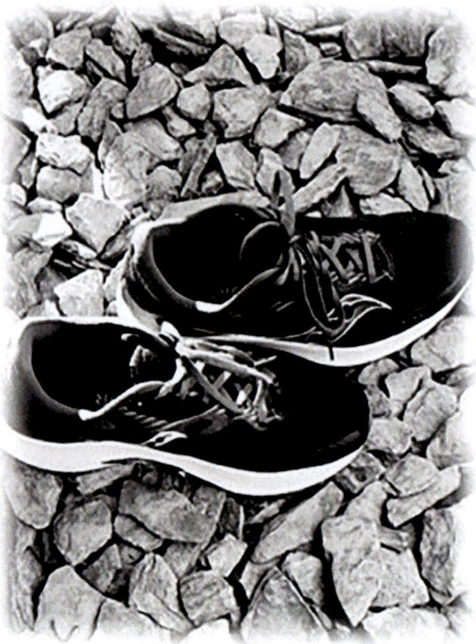

T-Shirt Thought

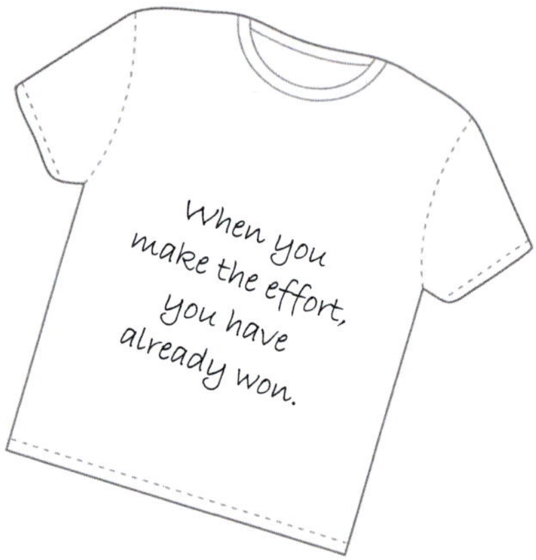

I am grateful; I am sympathetic

I am understanding; I am positive everyday

I am strong; I am dependable

I am honest; I am trustworthy

I will express my gratitude to the universe every day for all that I have and all that I am.

End of Day

A great attitude can change your mindset every day in every way...so it is worth the effort.

CONTEMPLATION

I am cared for; I am loved

I am intelligent; I am talented

I am accomplished; I am appreciated

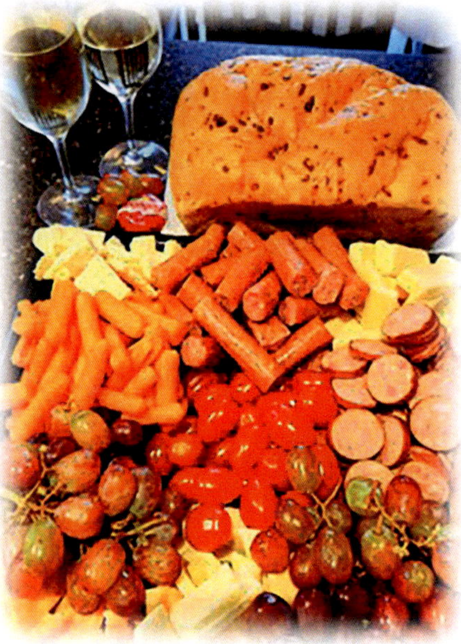

T-Shirt Thought

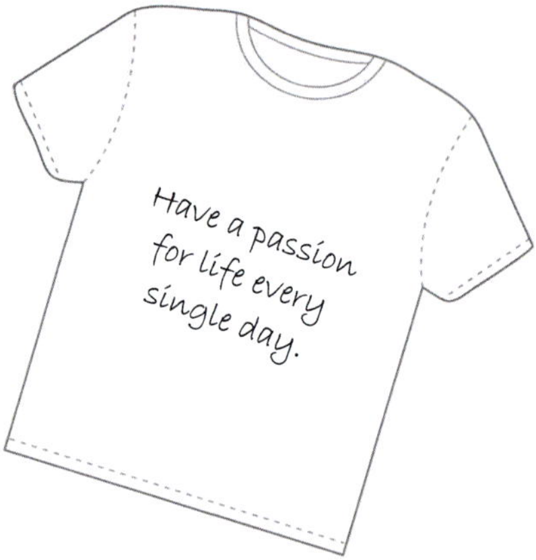

I am grateful; I am sympathetic

I am understanding; I am positive everyday

I am strong; I am dependable

I am honest; I am trustworthy

I will express my gratitude to the universe every day for all that I have and all that I am.

End of Day

When you look back at where you came from, how can you help but smile?

CONTEMPLATION

I am cared for; I am loved

I am intelligent; I am talented

I am accomplished; I am appreciated

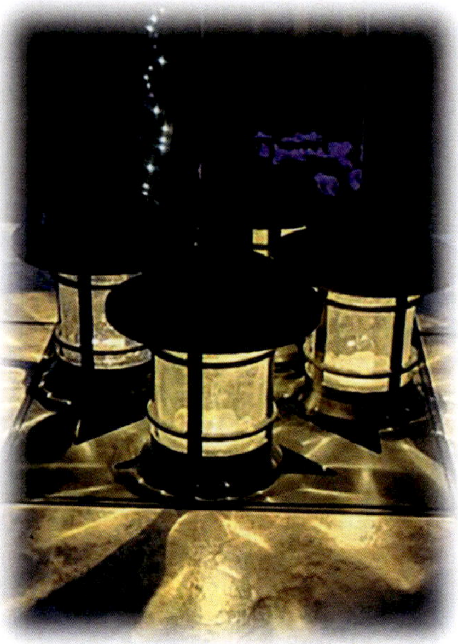

T-Shirt Thought

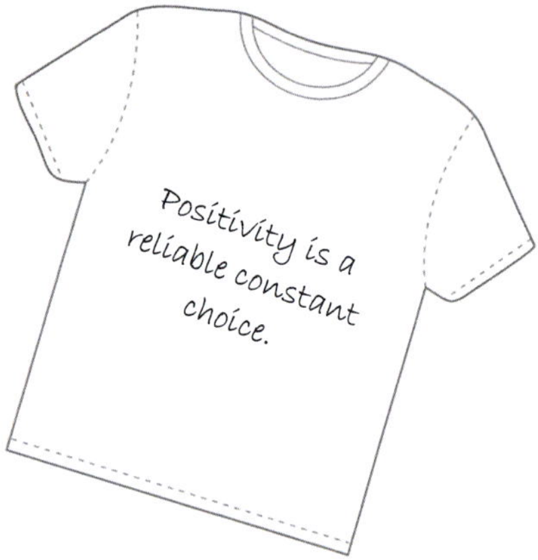

I am grateful; I am sympathetic

I am understanding; I am positive everyday

I am strong; I am dependable

I am honest; I am trustworthy

I will express my gratitude to the universe every day for all that I have and all that I am.

End of Day

No matter what it takes to turn the day around, it's always, always worth the effort.

CONTEMPLATION

I am cared for; I am loved

I am intelligent; I am talented

I am accomplished; I am appreciated

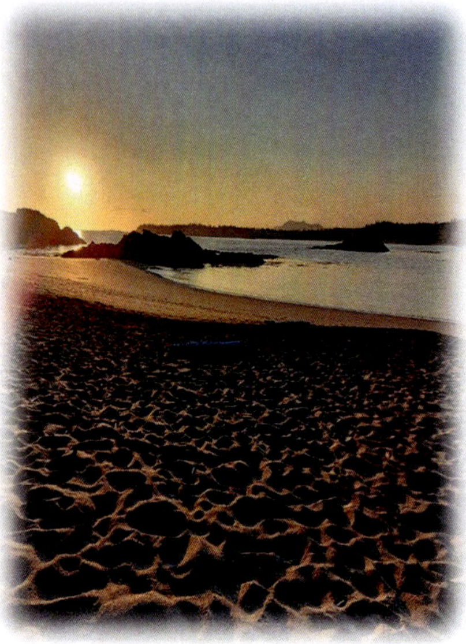

T-Shirt Thought

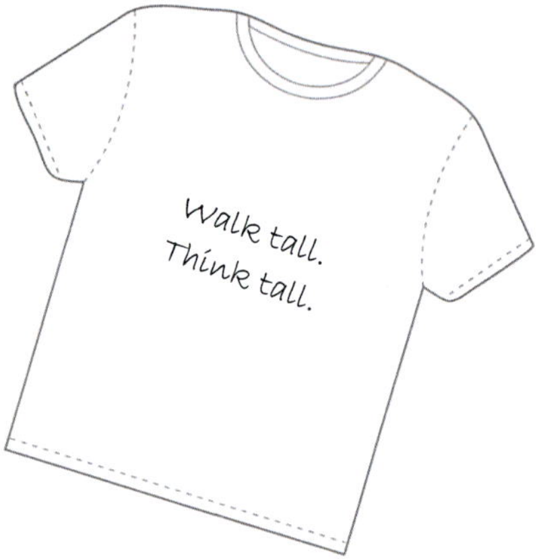

I am grateful; I am sympathetic

I am understanding; I am positive everyday

I am strong; I am dependable

I am honest; I am trustworthy

I will express my gratitude to the universe every day for all that I have and all that I am.

End of Day

Hard work is so much more rewarding than taking the easy way.

CONTEMPLATION

I am cared for; I am loved

I am intelligent; I am talented

I am accomplished; I am appreciated

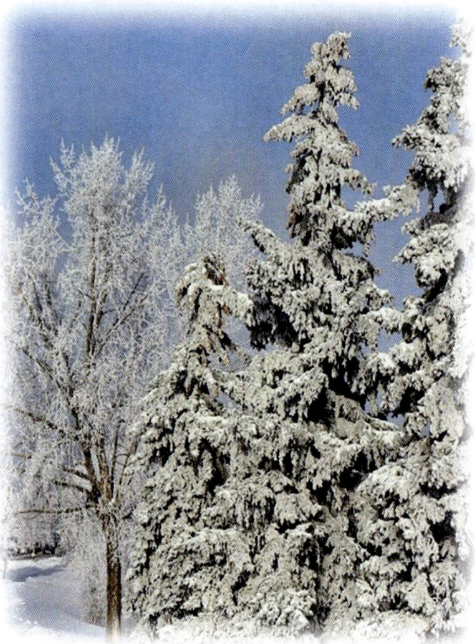

T-Shirt Thought

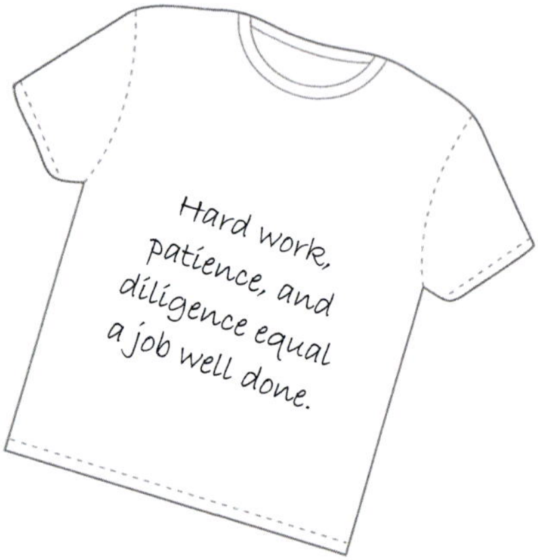

I am grateful; I am sympathetic

I am understanding; I am positive everyday

I am strong; I am dependable

I am honest; I am trustworthy

I will express my gratitude to the universe every day for all that I have and all that I am.

End of Day

Time wasted procrastinating is greater than the time spent on the task itself.

CONTEMPLATION

I am cared for; I am loved

I am intelligent; I am talented

I am accomplished; I am appreciated

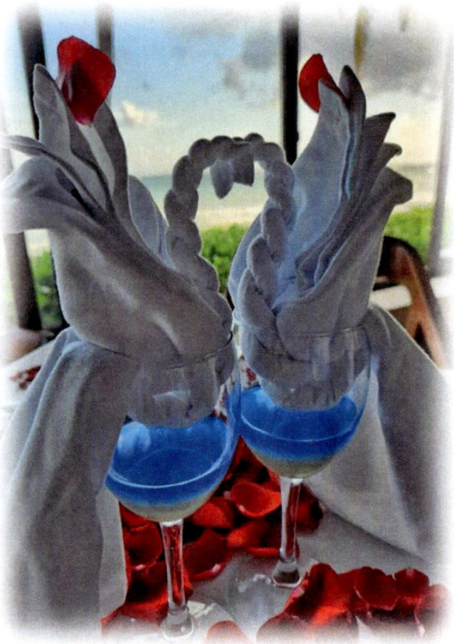

T-Shirt Thought

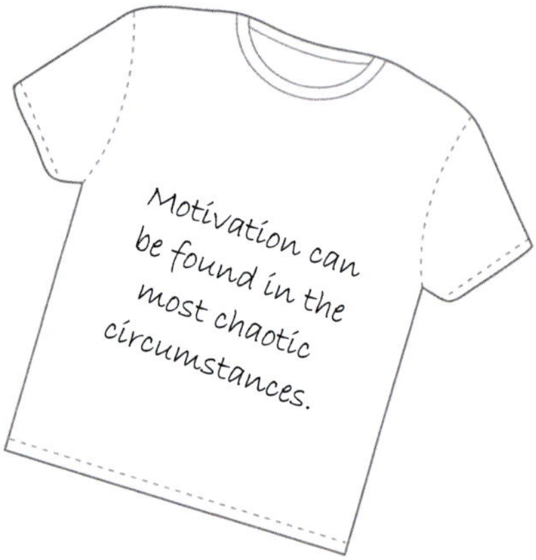

I am grateful; I am sympathetic

I am understanding; I am positive everyday

I am strong; I am dependable

I am honest; I am trustworthy

I will express my gratitude to the universe every day for all that I have and all that I am.

End of Day

The most difficult positive moment to find is the one most valuable.

CONTEMPLATION

I am cared for; I am loved

I am intelligent; I am talented

I am accomplished; I am appreciated

T-Shirt Thought

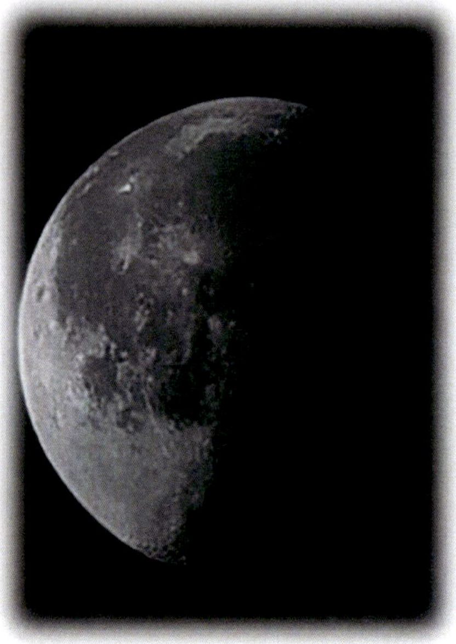

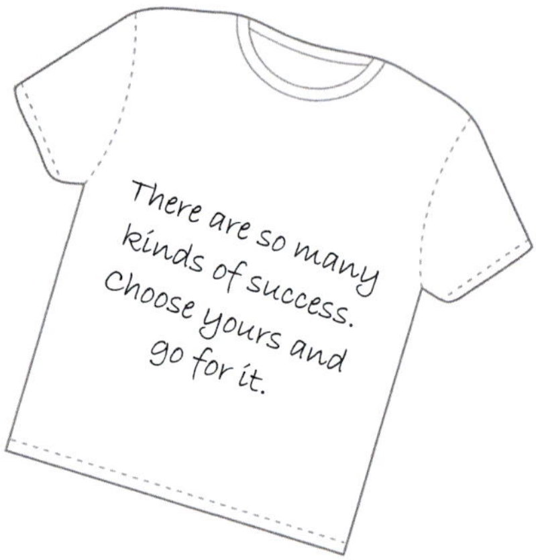

I am grateful; I am sympathetic

I am understanding; I am positive everyday

I am strong; I am dependable

I am honest; I am trustworthy

I will express my gratitude to the universe every day for all that I have and all that I am.

End of Day

Our strength is the most obvious in the way we handle setbacks.

CONTEMPLATION

I am cared for; I am loved

I am intelligent; I am talented

I am accomplished; I am appreciated

T-Shirt Thought

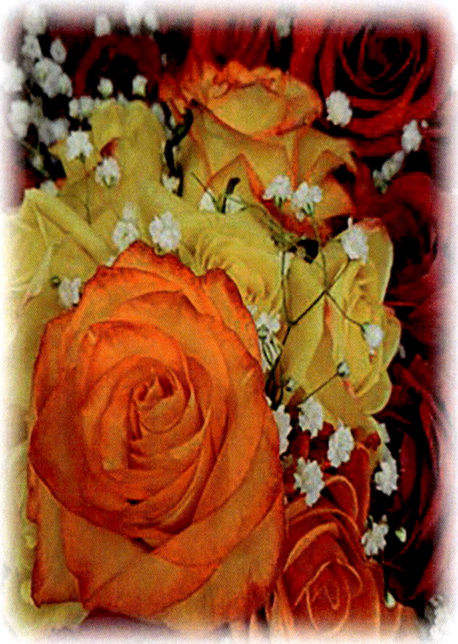

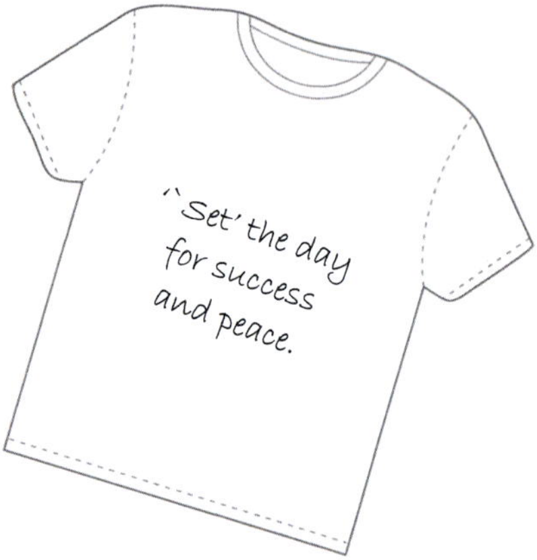

I am grateful; I am sympathetic

I am understanding; I am positive everyday

I am strong; I am dependable

I am honest; I am trustworthy

I will express my gratitude to the universe every day for all that I have and all that I am.

End of Day

When you collect all the little victories, before you know it, you have a huge achievement.

CONTEMPLATION

I am cared for; I am loved

I am intelligent; I am talented

I am accomplished; I am appreciated

T-Shirt Thought

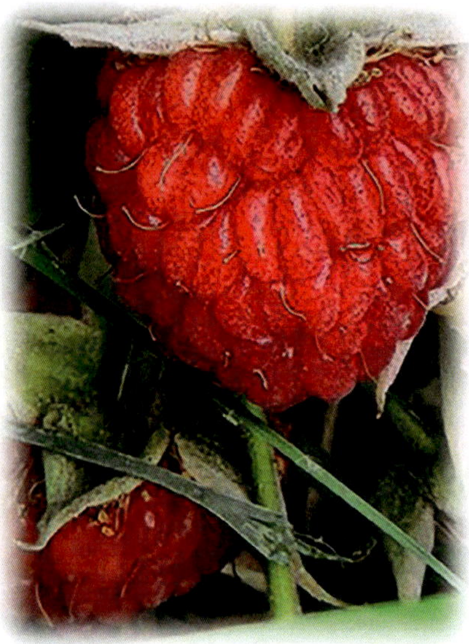

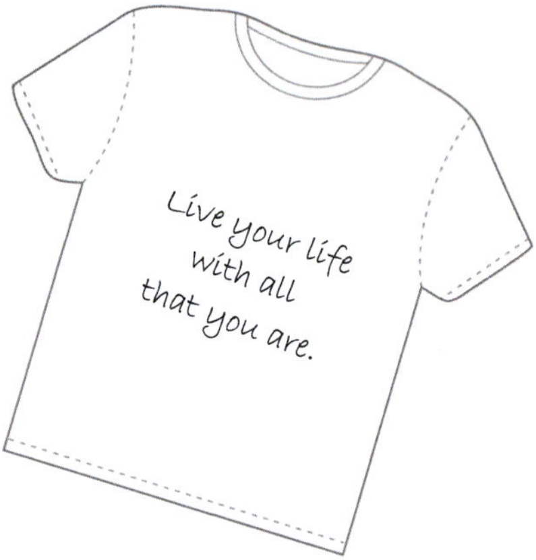

I am grateful; I am sympathetic

I am understanding; I am positive everyday

I am strong; I am dependable

I am honest; I am trustworthy

I will express my gratitude to the universe every day for all that I have and all that I am.

End of Day

Your mind has more control over your body than you realize.

CONTEMPLATION

I am cared for; I am loved

I am intelligent; I am talented

I am accomplished; I am appreciated

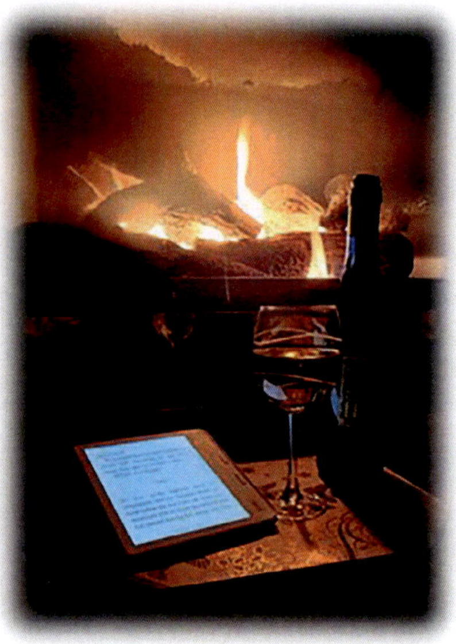

T-Shirt Thought

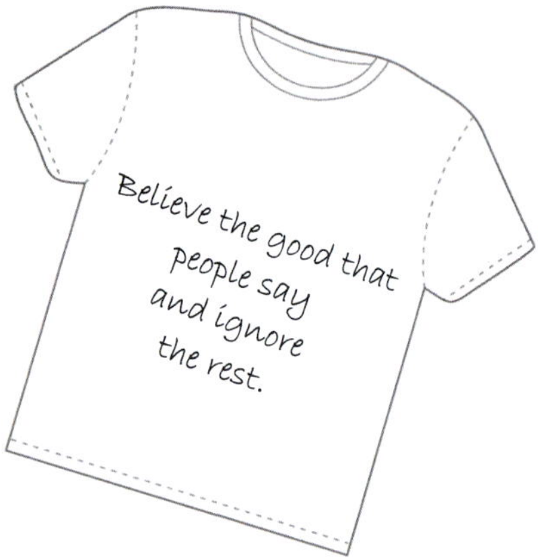

I am grateful; I am sympathetic

I am understanding; I am positive everyday

I am strong; I am dependable

I am honest; I am trustworthy

I will express my gratitude to the universe every day for all that I have and all that I am.

End of Day

Be gentle with yourself, you are the one who knows 'you' the best.

CONTEMPLATION

I am cared for; I am loved

I am intelligent; I am talented

I am accomplished; I am appreciated

T-Shirt Thought

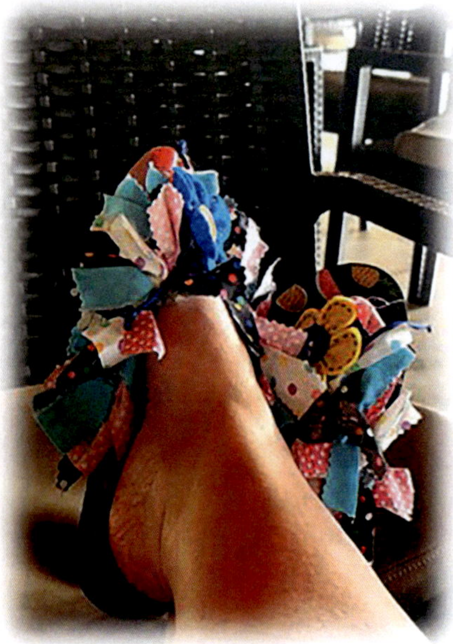

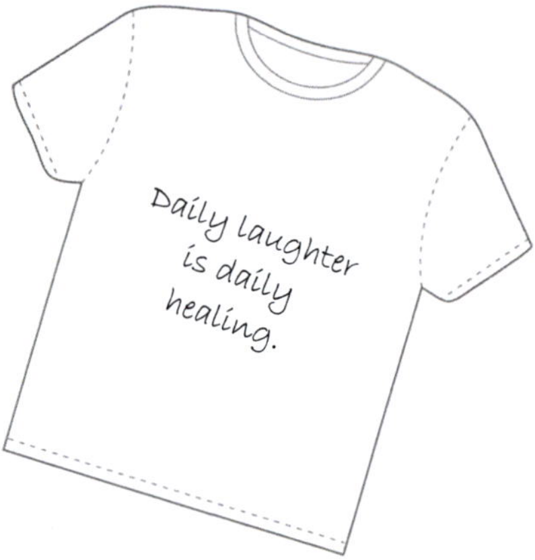

I am grateful; I am sympathetic

I am understanding; I am positive everyday

I am strong; I am dependable

I am honest; I am trustworthy

I will express my gratitude to the universe every day for all that I have and all that I am.

End of Day

Get up and put on a great attitude like you get dressed.

CONTEMPLATION

TOGETHER ON THE PATH

I am cared for; I am loved

I am intelligent; I am talented

I am accomplished; I am appreciated

T-Shirt Thought

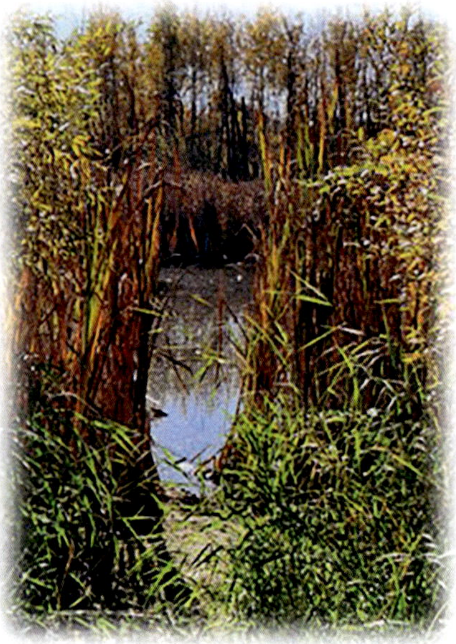

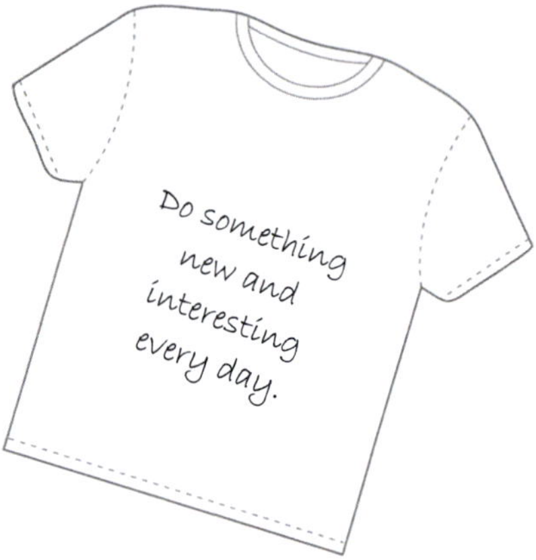

I am grateful; I am sympathetic

I am understanding; I am positive everyday

I am strong; I am dependable

I am honest; I am trustworthy

I will express my gratitude to the universe every day for all that I have and all that I am.

End of Day

When you do something you love, give it everything you have, and it will love you back.

CONTEMPLATION

I am cared for; I am loved

I am intelligent; I am talented

I am accomplished; I am appreciated

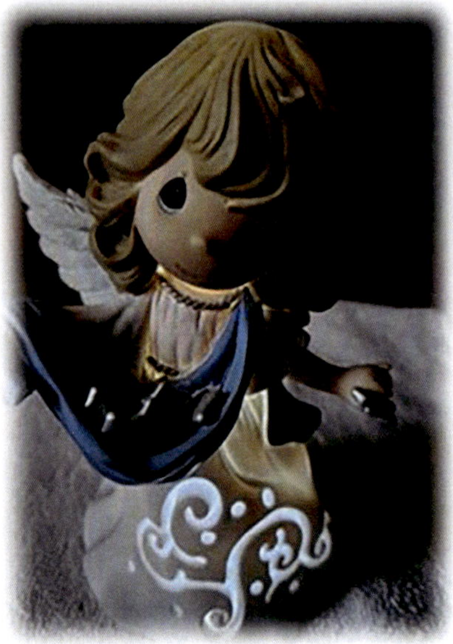

T-Shirt Thought

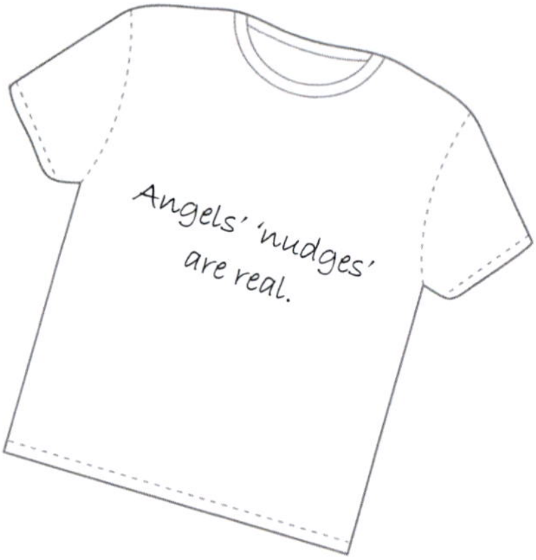

I am grateful; I am sympathetic

I am understanding; I am positive everyday

I am strong; I am dependable

I am honest; I am trustworthy

I will express my gratitude to the universe every day for all that I have and all that I am.

End of Day

'Off 'days are just reminders that no one is completely self- sufficient. Ask for help.

CONTEMPLATION

TOGETHER ON THE PATH

I am cared for; I am loved

I am intelligent; I am talented

I am accomplished; I am appreciated

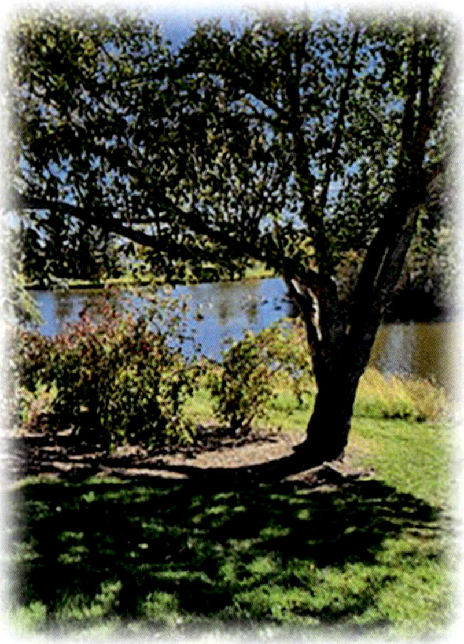

T-Shirt Thought

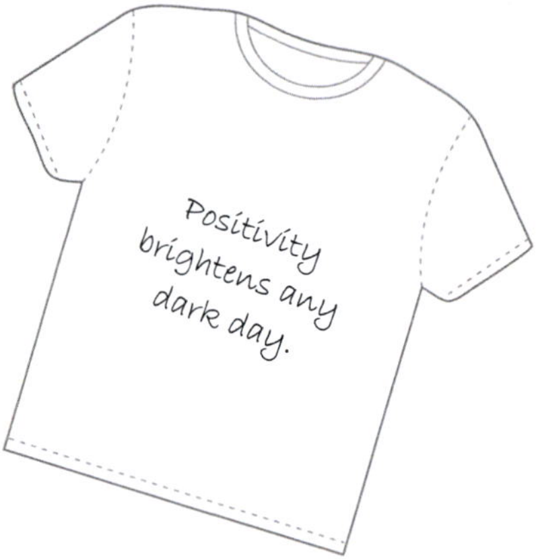

I am grateful; I am sympathetic

I am understanding; I am positive everyday

I am strong; I am dependable

I am honest; I am trustworthy

I will express my gratitude to the universe every day for all that I have and all that I am.

End of Day

A simple kind word can make you soar for the whole day, whether taken or given.

CONTEMPLATION

TOGETHER ON THE PATH

I am cared for; I am loved

I am intelligent; I am talented

I am accomplished; I am appreciated

T-Shirt Thought

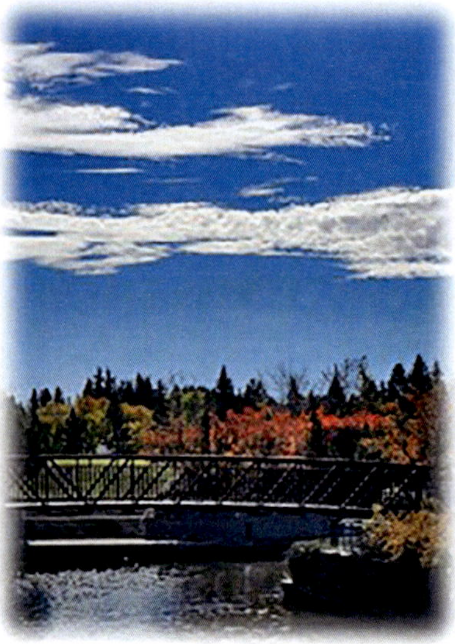

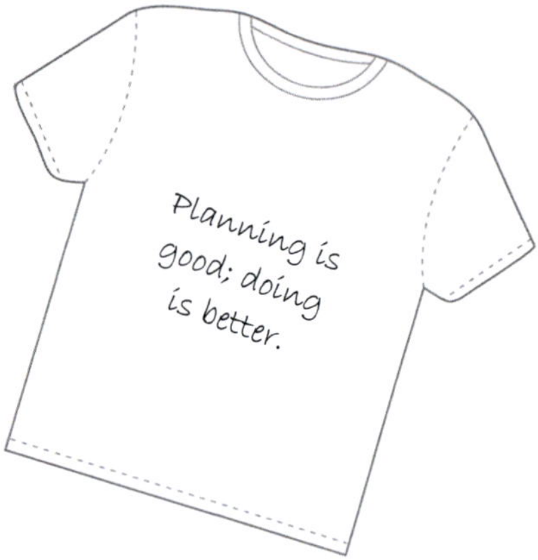

I am grateful; I am sympathetic

I am understanding; I am positive everyday

I am strong; I am dependable

I am honest; I am trustworthy

I will express my gratitude to the universe every day for all that I have and all that I am.

End of Day

When you organize your workspace, you renew your enthusiasm for the work.

CONTEMPLATION

I am cared for; I am loved

I am intelligent; I am talented

I am accomplished; I am appreciated

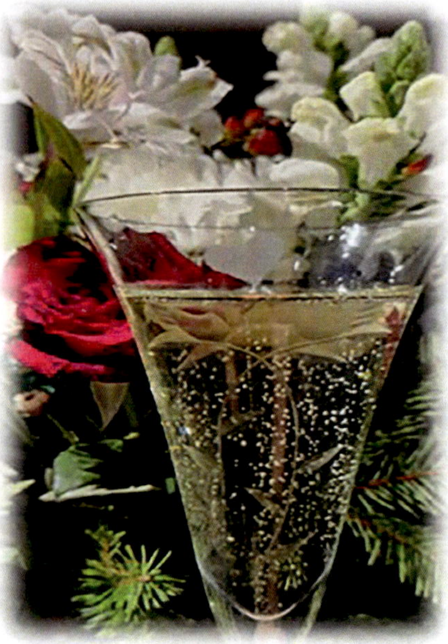

T-Shirt Thought

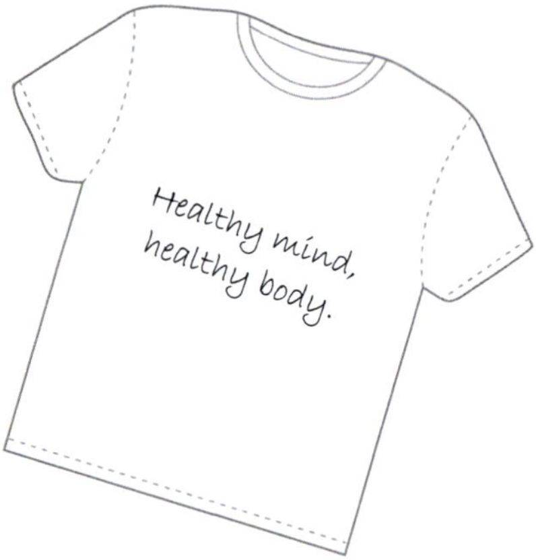

I am grateful; I am sympathetic

I am understanding; I am positive everyday

I am strong; I am dependable

I am honest; I am trustworthy

I will express my gratitude to the universe every day for all that I have and all that I am.

End of Day

Dirty hands are happy hands, so let's get dirty.

CONTEMPLATION

TOGETHER ON THE PATH

I am cared for; I am loved

I am intelligent; I am talented

I am accomplished; I am appreciated

T-Shirt Thought

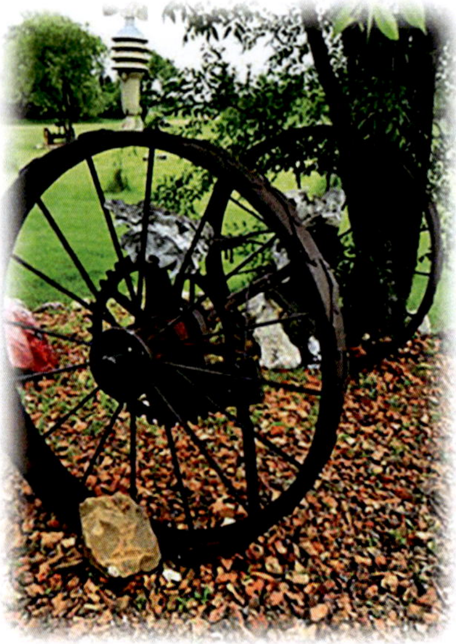

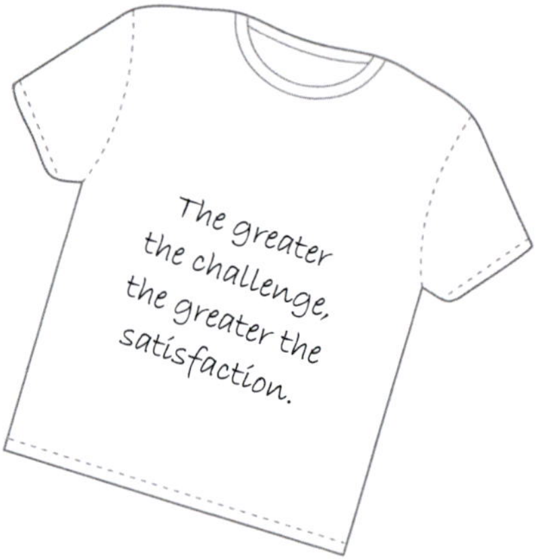

I am grateful; I am sympathetic

I am understanding; I am positive everyday

I am strong; I am dependable

I am honest; I am trustworthy

I will express my gratitude to the universe every day for all that I have and all that I am.

End of Day

Perseverance can solve so many problems. Just hang in there and make it work.

CONTEMPLATION

TOGETHER ON THE PATH

I am cared for; I am loved

I am intelligent; I am talented

I am accomplished; I am appreciated

T-Shirt Thought

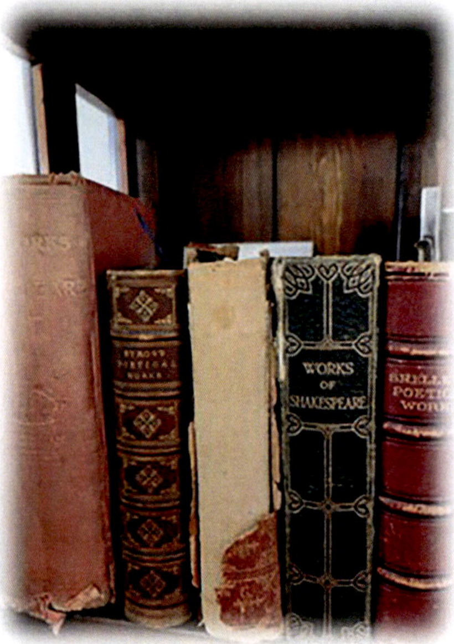

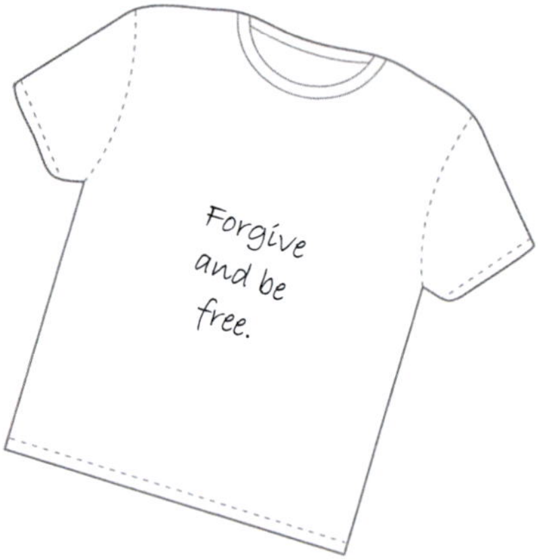

I am grateful; I am sympathetic

I am understanding; I am positive everyday

I am strong; I am dependable

I am honest; I am trustworthy

I will express my gratitude to the universe every day for all that I have and all that I am.

End of Day

Learning to forgive yourself is truly liberating.

CONTEMPLATION

I am cared for; I am loved

I am intelligent; I am talented

I am accomplished; I am appreciated

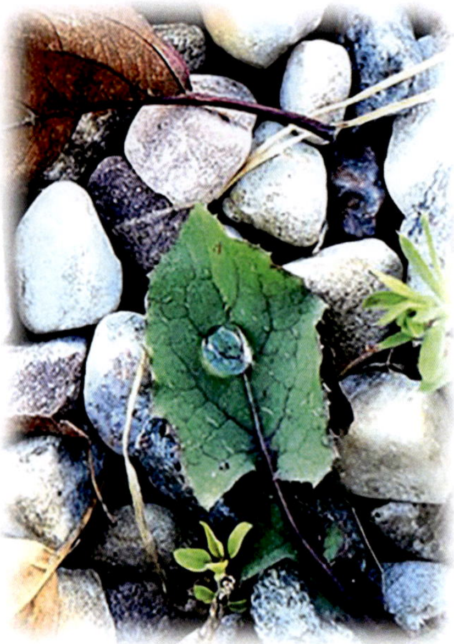

T-Shirt Thought

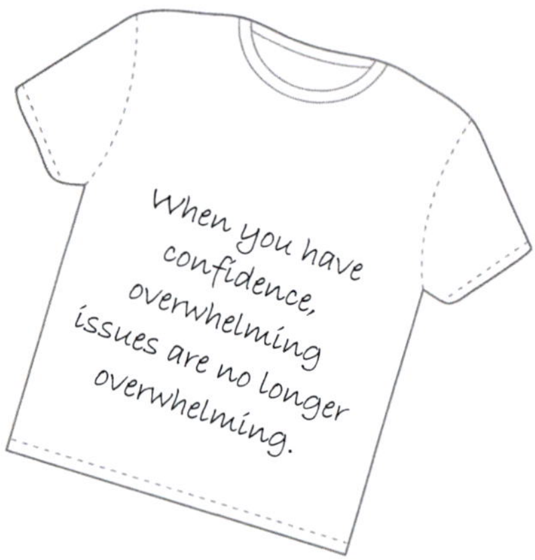

I am grateful; I am sympathetic

I am understanding; I am positive everyday

I am strong; I am dependable

I am honest; I am trustworthy

I will express my gratitude to the universe every day for all that I have and all that I am.

End of Day

If you are never challenged, you will never grow, so stare down that challenge and take a leap.

CONTEMPLATION

I am cared for; I am loved

I am intelligent; I am talented

I am accomplished; I am appreciated

T-Shirt Thought

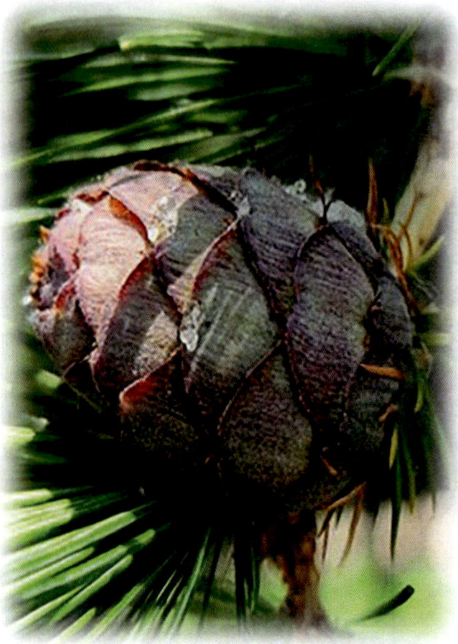

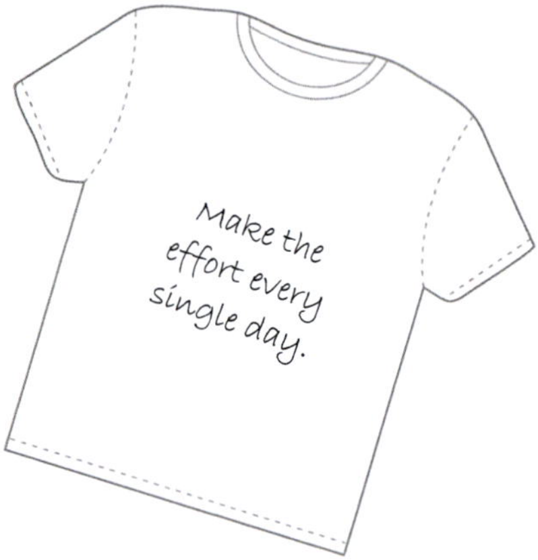

I am grateful; I am sympathetic

I am understanding; I am positive everyday

I am strong; I am dependable

I am honest; I am trustworthy

I will express my gratitude to the universe every day for all that I have and all that I am.

End of Day

A tough day does not mean an unsuccessful day.

CONTEMPLATION

I am cared for; I am loved

I am intelligent; I am talented

I am accomplished; I am appreciated

T-Shirt Thought

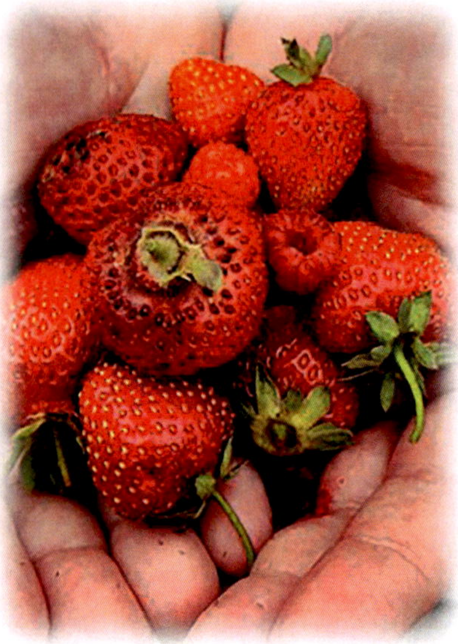

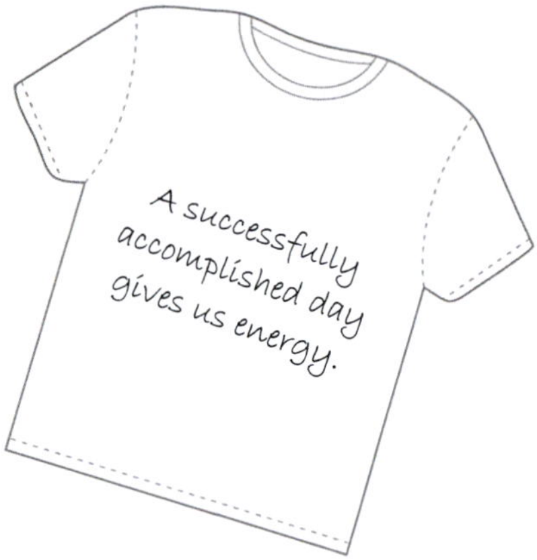

I am grateful; I am sympathetic

I am understanding; I am positive everyday

I am strong; I am dependable

I am honest; I am trustworthy

I will express my gratitude to the universe every day for all that I have and all that I am.

End of Day

Some days are extremely up. Some are extremely down. The important thing is to find the balance and believe you can do it.

CONTEMPLATION

I am cared for; I am loved

I am intelligent; I am talented

I am accomplished; I am appreciated

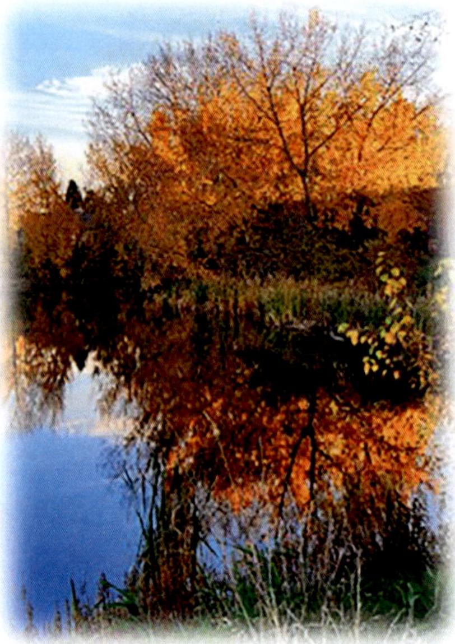

T-Shirt Thought

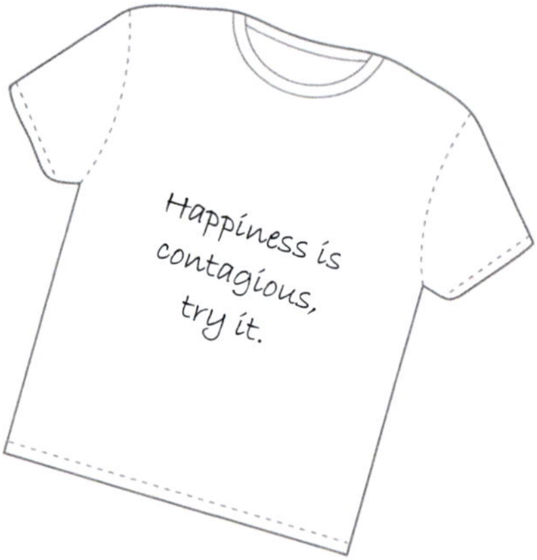

I am grateful; I am sympathetic

I am understanding; I am positive everyday

I am strong; I am dependable

I am honest; I am trustworthy

I will express my gratitude to the universe every day for all that I have and all that I am.

End of Day

When you find the right music, you find the right mindset.

CONTEMPLATION

TOGETHER ON THE PATH

I am cared for; I am loved

I am intelligent; I am talented

I am accomplished; I am appreciated

T-Shirt Thought

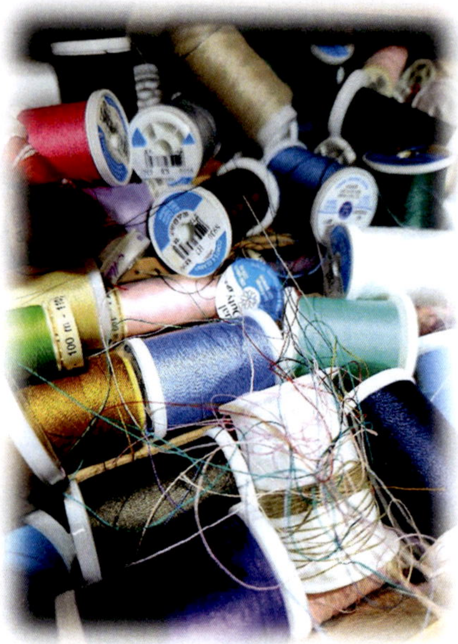

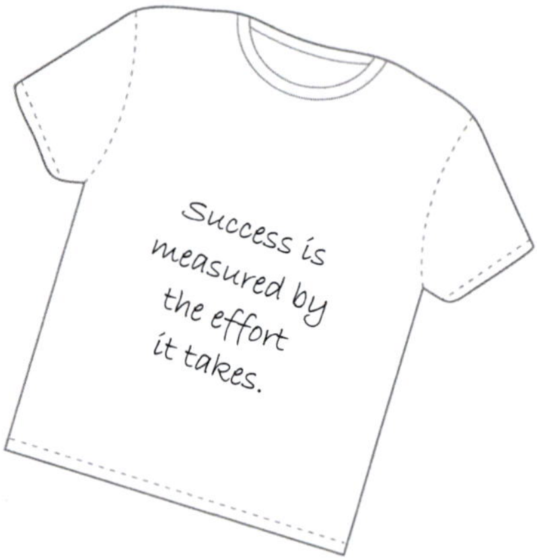

I am grateful; I am sympathetic

I am understanding; I am positive everyday

I am strong; I am dependable

I am honest; I am trustworthy

I will express my gratitude to the universe every day for all that I have and all that I am.

End of Day

Only look back when looking back pushes you forward.

CONTEMPLATION

TOGETHER ON THE PATH

I am cared for; I am loved

I am intelligent; I am talented

I am accomplished; I am appreciated

T-Shirt Thought

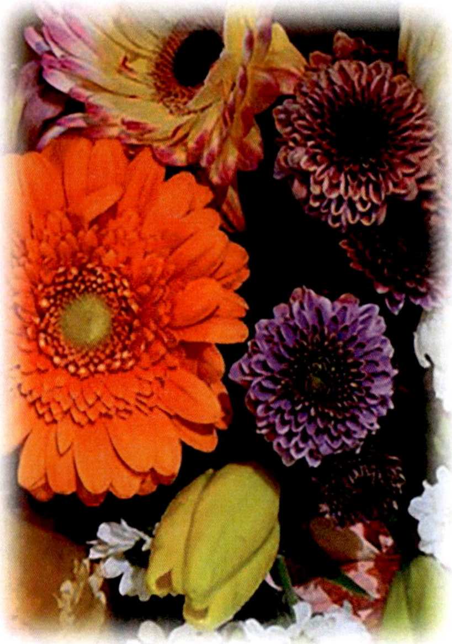

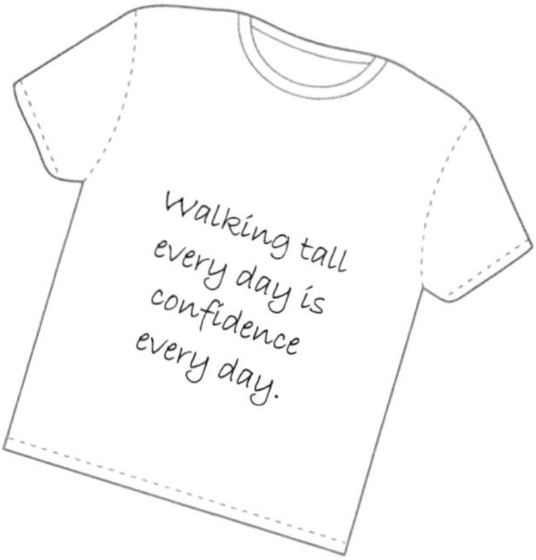

I am grateful; I am sympathetic

I am understanding; I am positive everyday

I am strong; I am dependable

I am honest; I am trustworthy

I will express my gratitude to the universe every day for all that I have and all that I am.

End of Day

A physical limitation does not mean a mental limitation; keep going.

CONTEMPLATION

I am cared for; I am loved

I am intelligent; I am talented

I am accomplished; I am appreciated

T-Shirt Thought

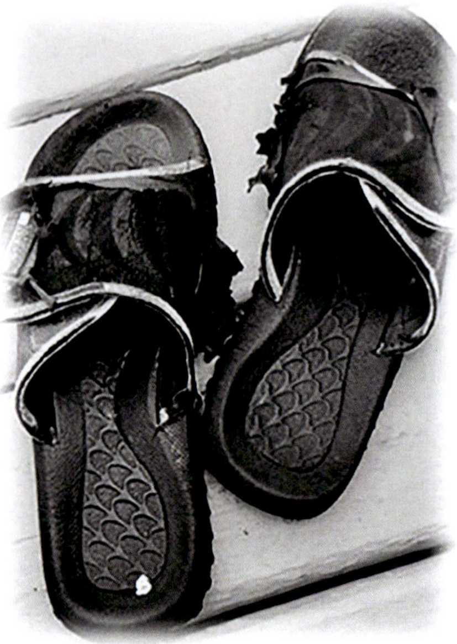

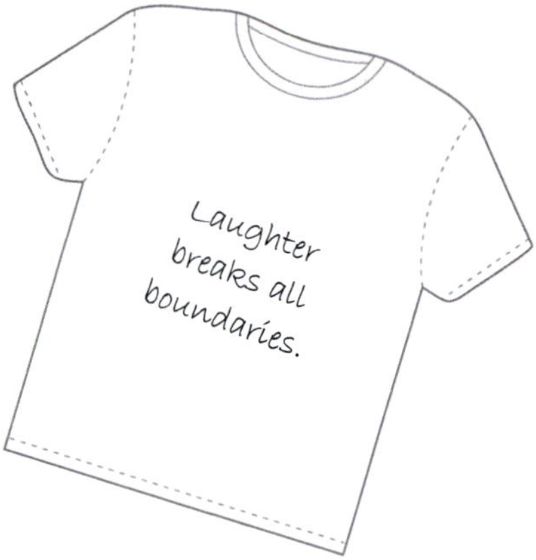

I am grateful; I am sympathetic

I am understanding; I am positive everyday

I am strong; I am dependable

I am honest; I am trustworthy

I will express my gratitude to the universe every day for all that I have and all that I am.

End of Day

A day that starts with humor ends with a smile.

CONTEMPLATION

I am cared for; I am loved

I am intelligent; I am talented

I am accomplished; I am appreciated

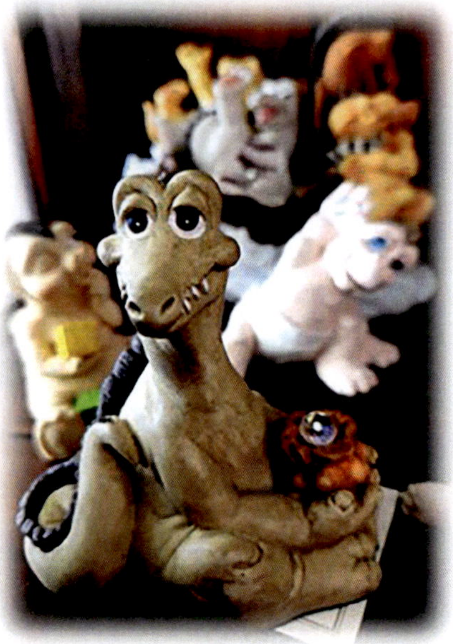

T-Shirt Thought

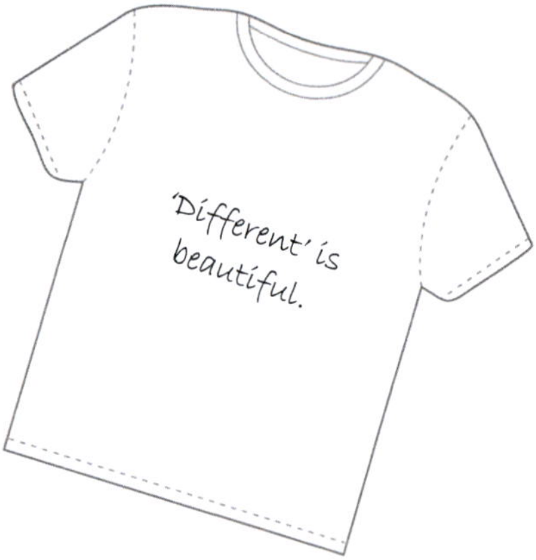

I am grateful; I am sympathetic

I am understanding; I am positive everyday

I am strong; I am dependable

I am honest; I am trustworthy

I will express my gratitude to the universe every day for all that I have and all that I am.

End of Day

So many different kinds of people in the world...like beautiful bouquets of different flowers.

CONTEMPLATION

I am cared for; I am loved

I am intelligent; I am talented

I am accomplished; I am appreciated

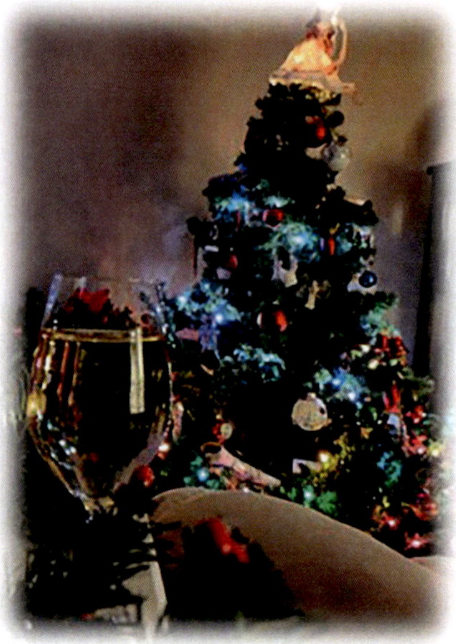

T-Shirt Thought

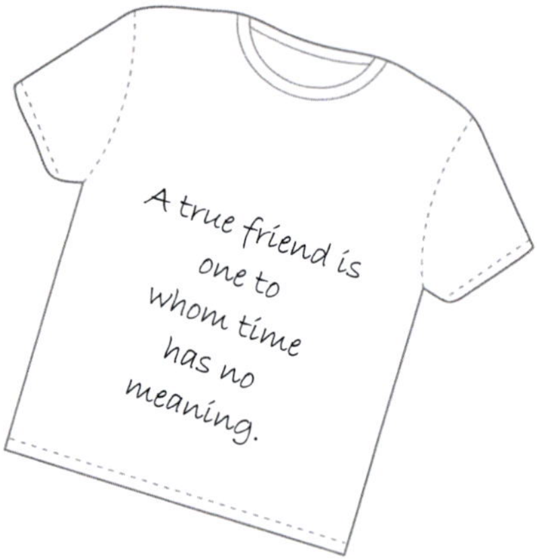

I am grateful; I am sympathetic

I am understanding; I am positive everyday

I am strong; I am dependable

I am honest; I am trustworthy

I will express my gratitude to the universe every day for all that I have and all that I am.

End of Day

Never be afraid to ask for help. You will undoubtedly help someone else in time.

CONTEMPLATION

I am cared for; I am loved

I am intelligent; I am talented

I am accomplished; I am appreciated

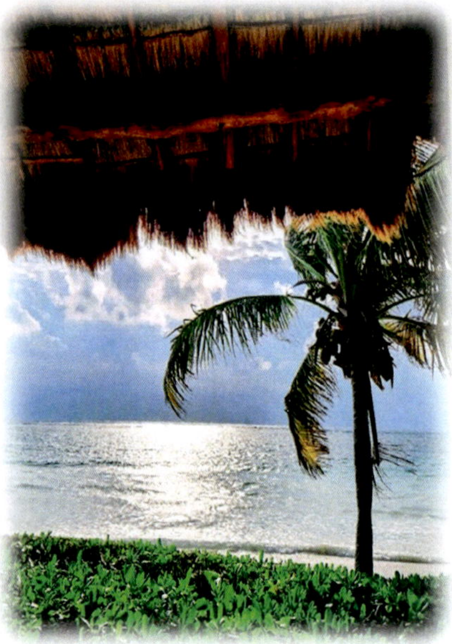

T-Shirt Thought

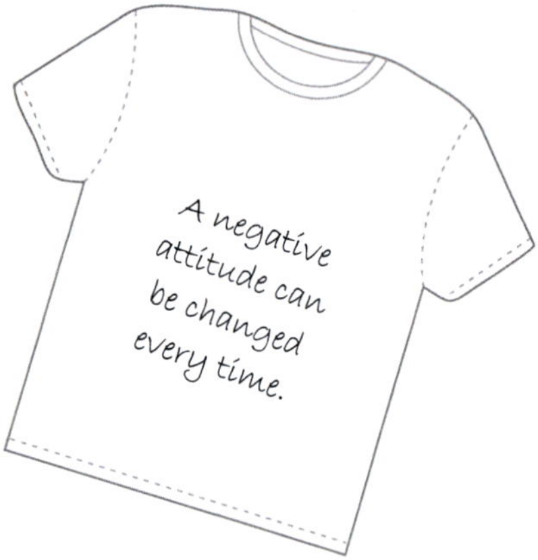

I am grateful; I am sympathetic

I am understanding; I am positive everyday

I am strong; I am dependable

I am honest; I am trustworthy

I will express my gratitude to the universe every day for all that I have and all that I am.

End of Day

A bad day can be turned around completely by one positive event.

CONTEMPLATION

I am cared for; I am loved

I am intelligent; I am talented

I am accomplished; I am appreciated

T-Shirt Thought

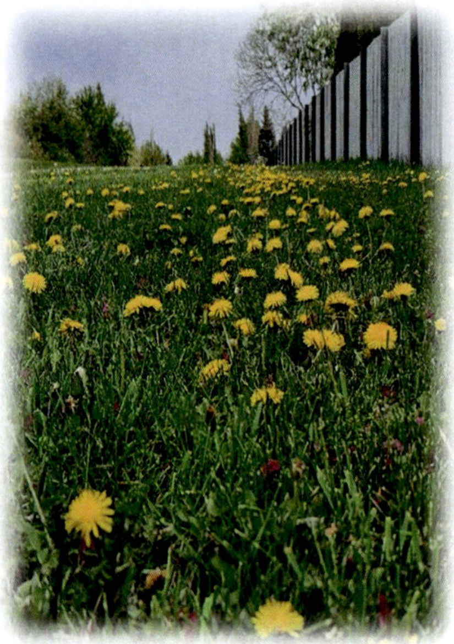

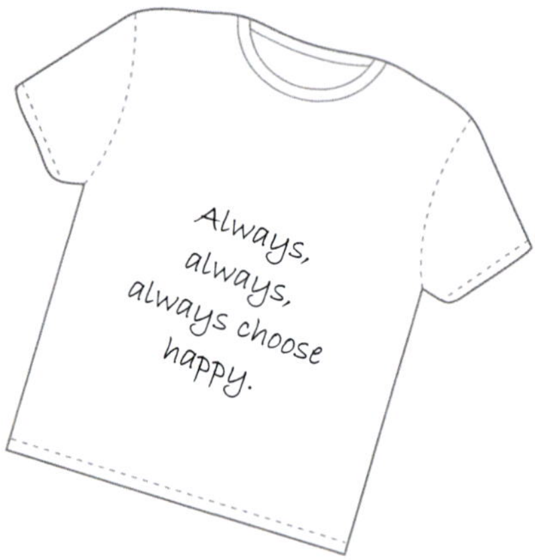

I am grateful; I am sympathetic

I am understanding; I am positive everyday

I am strong; I am dependable

I am honest; I am trustworthy

I will express my gratitude to the universe every day for all that I have and all that I am.

End of Day

The attitude you choose is the attitude you spread, so spread happiness.

CONTEMPLATION

I am cared for; I am loved

I am intelligent; I am talented

I am accomplished; I am appreciated

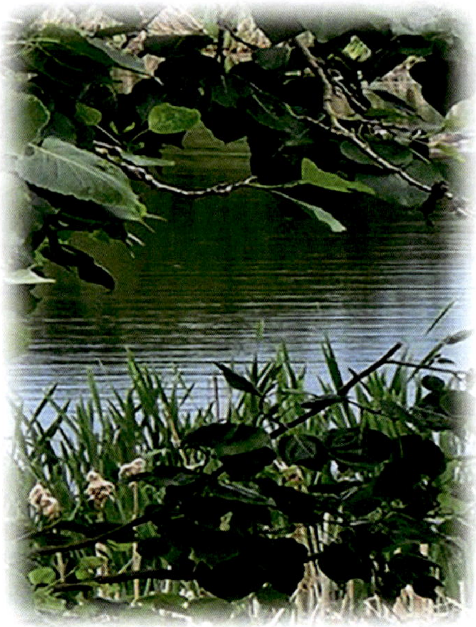

T-Shirt Thought

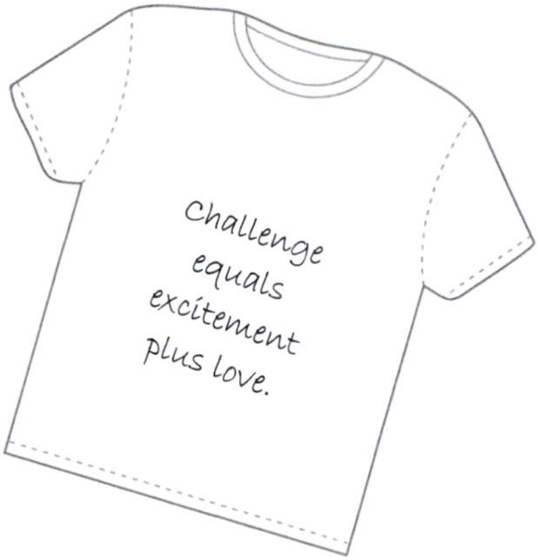

I am grateful; I am sympathetic

I am understanding; I am positive everyday

I am strong; I am dependable

I am honest; I am trustworthy

I will express my gratitude to the universe every day for all that I have and all that I am.

End of Day

Stress is just part of the excitement.

CONTEMPLATION

I am cared for; I am loved

I am intelligent; I am talented

I am accomplished; I am appreciated

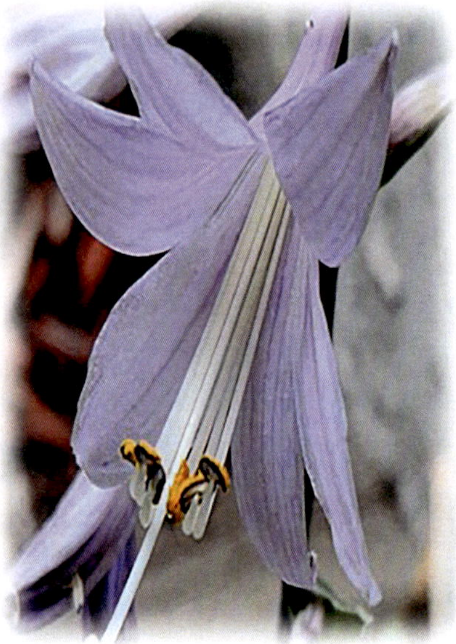

T-Shirt Thought

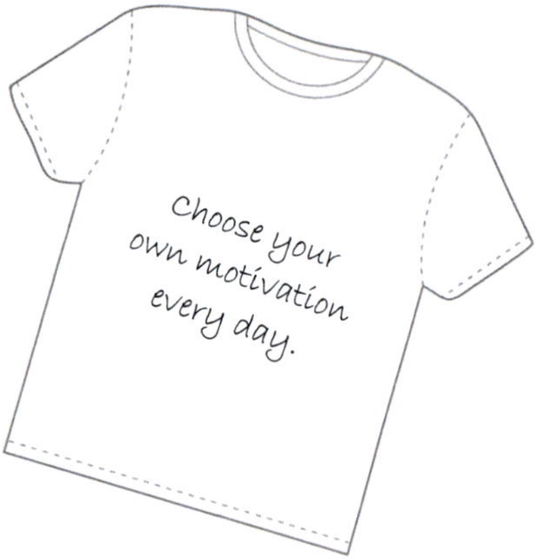

I am grateful; I am sympathetic

I am understanding; I am positive everyday

I am strong; I am dependable

I am honest; I am trustworthy

I will express my gratitude to the universe every day for all that I have and all that I am.

End of Day

'Inspired' and 'inspiring' are micro-thoughts apart.

CONTEMPLATION

I am cared for; I am loved

I am intelligent; I am talented

I am accomplished; I am appreciated

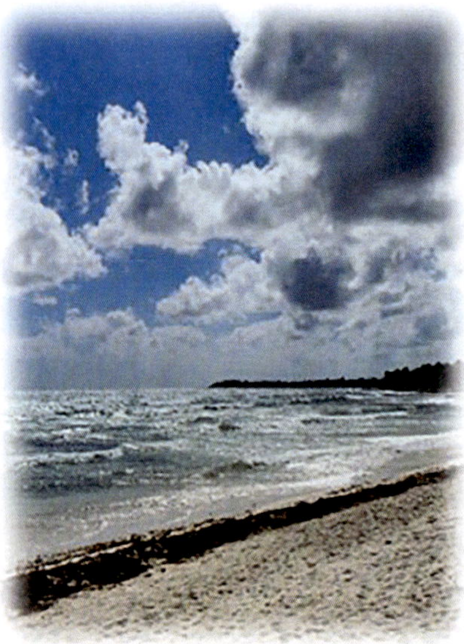

T-Shirt Thought

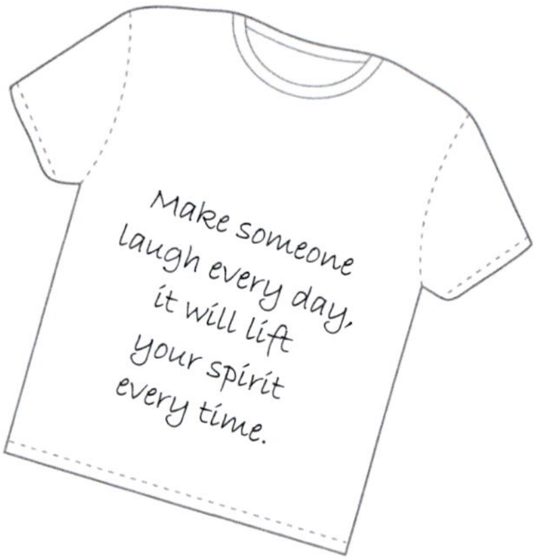

I am grateful; I am sympathetic

I am understanding; I am positive everyday

I am strong; I am dependable

I am honest; I am trustworthy

I will express my gratitude to the universe every day for all that I have and all that I am.

End of Day

Being with friends for fun and laughter is so soul- soothing.

CONTEMPLATION

I am cared for; I am loved

I am intelligent; I am talented

I am accomplished; I am appreciated

T-Shirt Thought

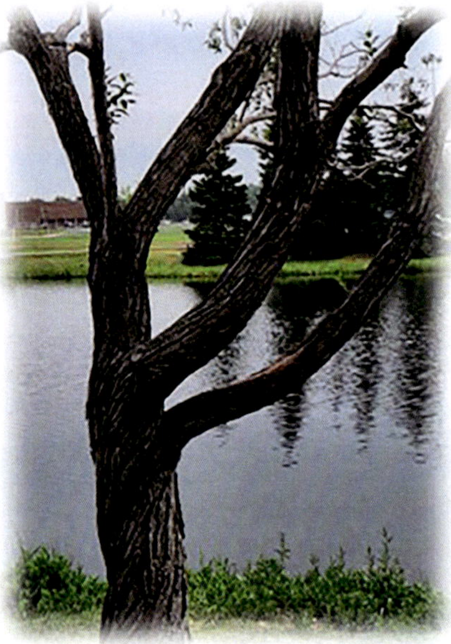

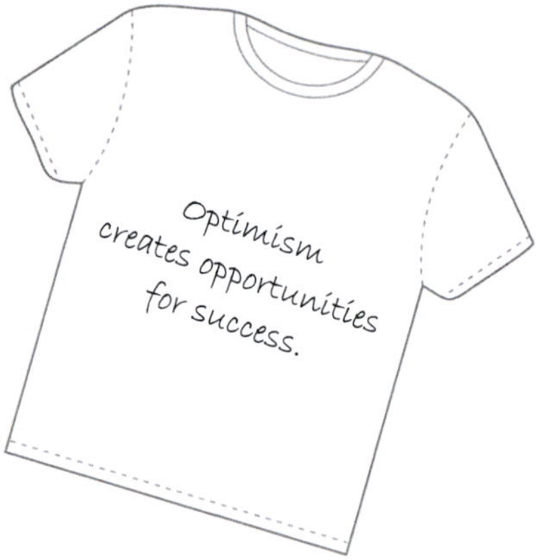

I am grateful; I am sympathetic

I am understanding; I am positive everyday

I am strong; I am dependable

I am honest; I am trustworthy

I will express my gratitude to the universe every day for all that I have and all that I am.

End of Day

The beginning of a new exciting project is a truly challenging adventure.

CONTEMPLATION

I am cared for; I am loved

I am intelligent; I am talented

I am accomplished; I am appreciated

T-Shirt Thought

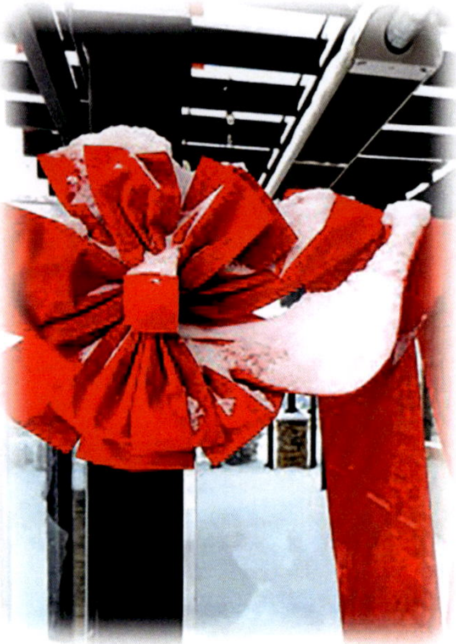

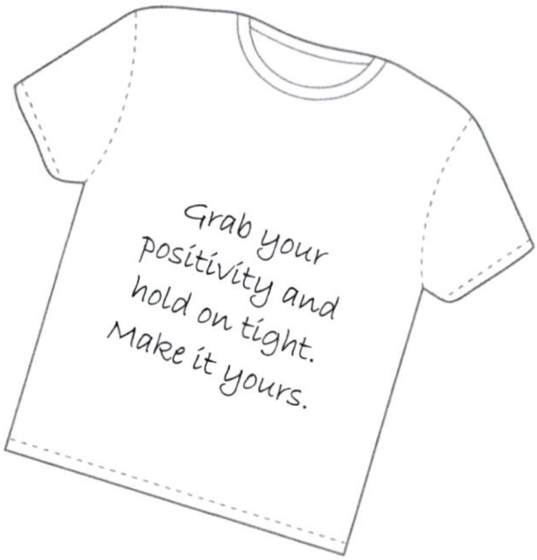

I am grateful; I am sympathetic

I am understanding; I am positive everyday

I am strong; I am dependable

I am honest; I am trustworthy

I will express my gratitude to the universe every day for all that I have and all that I am.

End of Day

A positive mindset change can be habit forming and easier with every effort.

CONTEMPLATION

TOGETHER ON THE PATH

I am cared for; I am loved

I am intelligent; I am talented

I am accomplished; I am appreciated

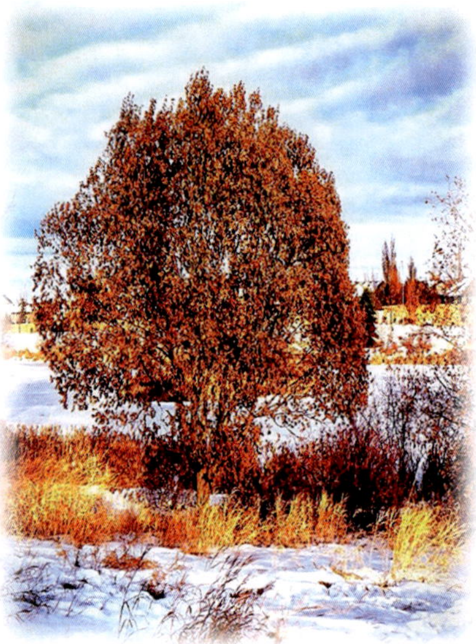

T-Shirt Thought

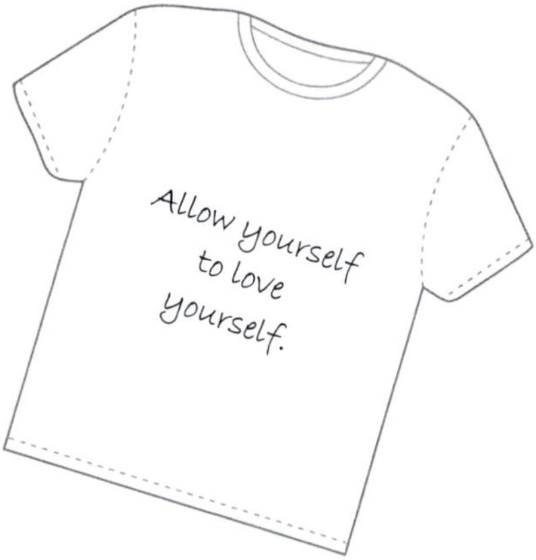

I am grateful; I am sympathetic

I am understanding; I am positive everyday

I am strong; I am dependable

I am honest; I am trustworthy

I will express my gratitude to the universe every day for all that I have and all that I am.

End of Day

A lazy day must be treated as a day of peace and recovery, not a day without value.

CONTEMPLATION

I am cared for; I am loved

I am intelligent; I am talented

I am accomplished; I am appreciated

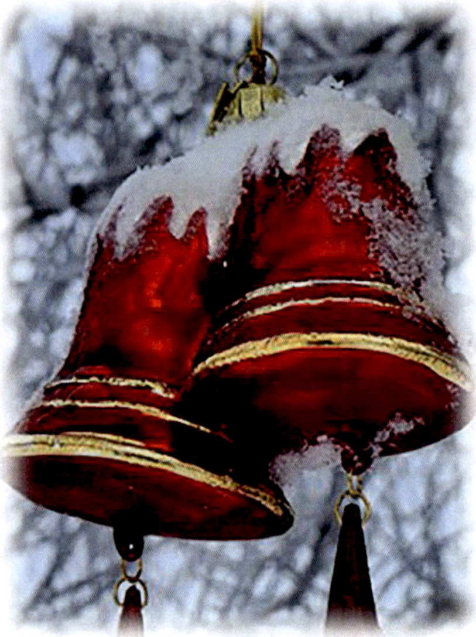

T-Shirt Thought

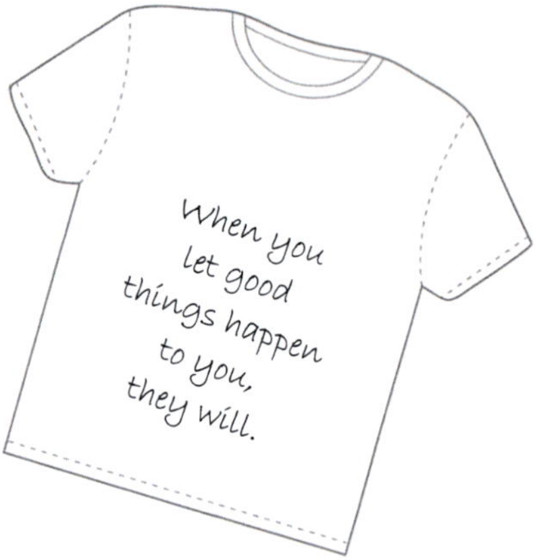

I am grateful; I am sympathetic

I am understanding; I am positive everyday

I am strong; I am dependable

I am honest; I am trustworthy

I will express my gratitude to the universe every day for all that I have and all that I am.

End of Day

Dream it, believe it, make it real, you're the only one who can.

CONTEMPLATION

TOGETHER ON THE PATH

I am cared for; I am loved

I am intelligent; I am talented

I am accomplished; I am appreciated

T-Shirt Thought

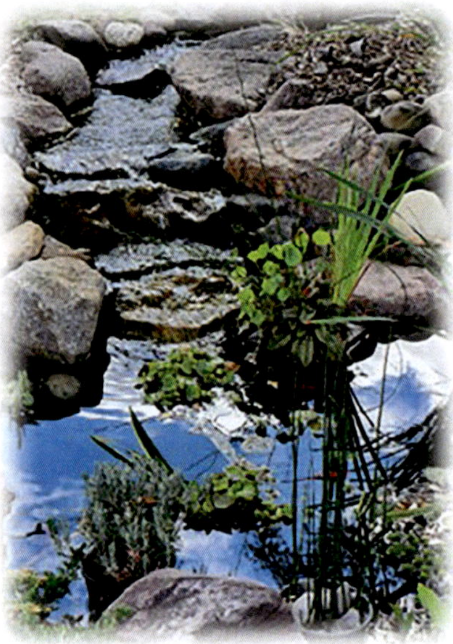

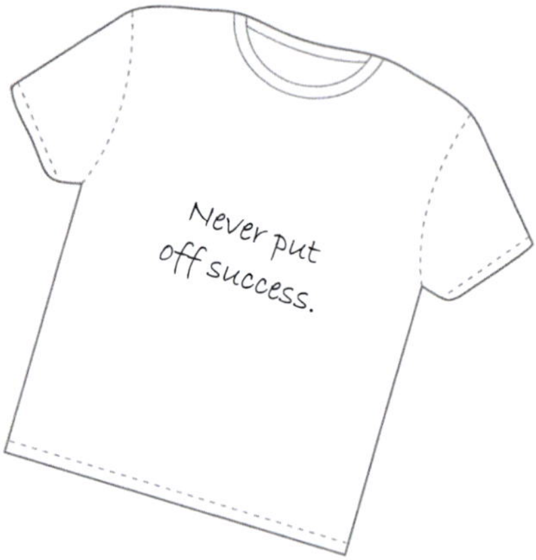

I am grateful; I am sympathetic

I am understanding; I am positive everyday

I am strong; I am dependable

I am honest; I am trustworthy

I will express my gratitude to the universe every day for all that I have and all that I am.

End of Day

Any day I can make someone laugh is a satisfying day no matter what else happens.

CONTEMPLATION

TOGETHER ON THE PATH

I am cared for; I am loved

I am intelligent; I am talented

I am accomplished; I am appreciated

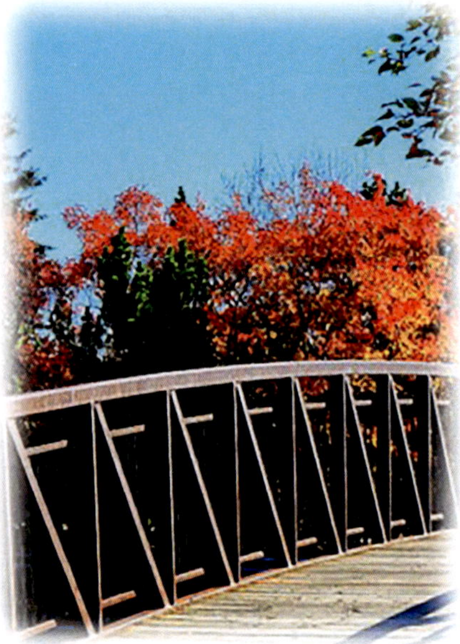

T-Shirt Thought

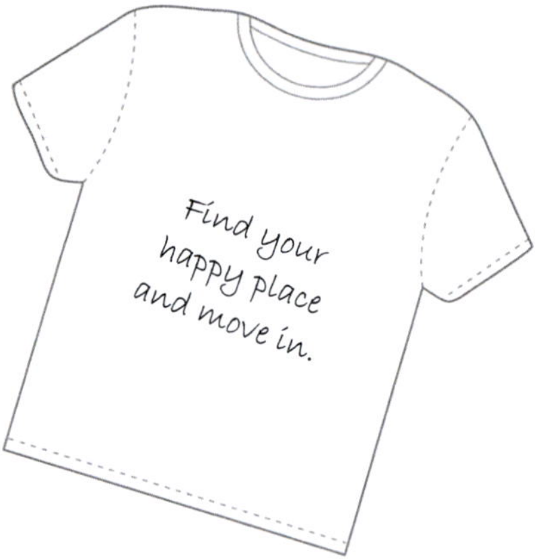

I am grateful; I am sympathetic

I am understanding; I am positive everyday

I am strong; I am dependable

I am honest; I am trustworthy

I will express my gratitude to the universe every day for all that I have and all that I am.

End of Day

Never assume the good days will continue. Assume you will get through them in peace.

CONTEMPLATION

I am cared for; I am loved

I am intelligent; I am talented

I am accomplished; I am appreciated

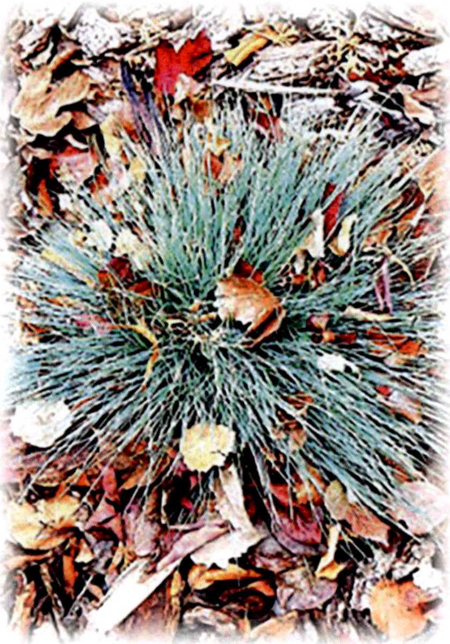

T-Shirt Thought

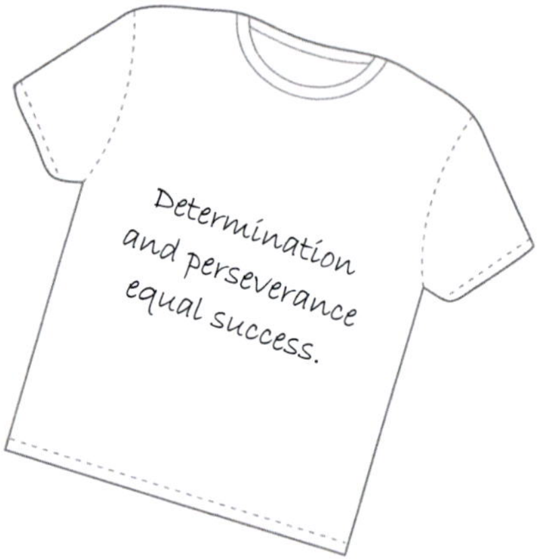

I am grateful; I am sympathetic

I am understanding; I am positive everyday

I am strong; I am dependable

I am honest; I am trustworthy

I will express my gratitude to the universe every day for all that I have and all that I am.

End of Day

So many little accomplishments, so many little victories.

CONTEMPLATION

TOGETHER ON THE PATH

I am cared for; I am loved

I am intelligent; I am talented

I am accomplished; I am appreciated

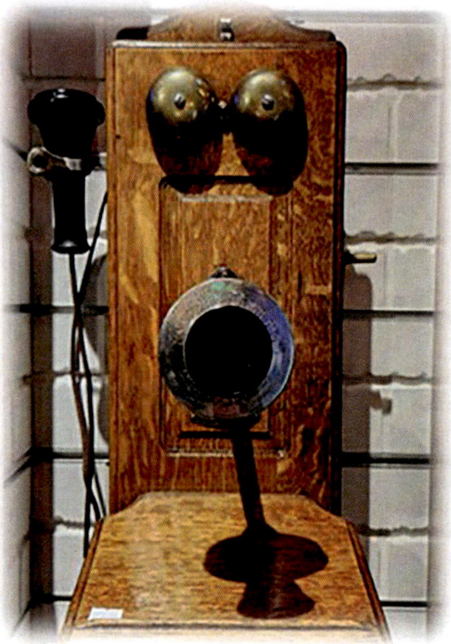

T-Shirt Thought

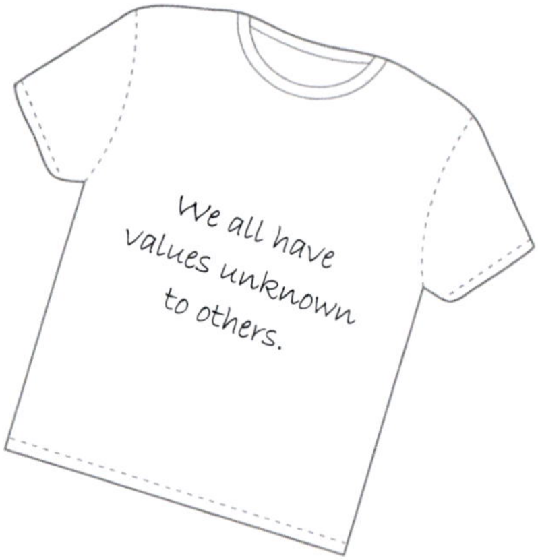

I am grateful; I am sympathetic

I am understanding; I am positive everyday

I am strong; I am dependable

I am honest; I am trustworthy

I will express my gratitude to the universe every day for all that I have and all that I am.

End of Day

The sooner we see our own value in our own eyes; the sooner we see it in others.

CONTEMPLATION

I am cared for; I am loved

I am intelligent; I am talented

I am accomplished; I am appreciated

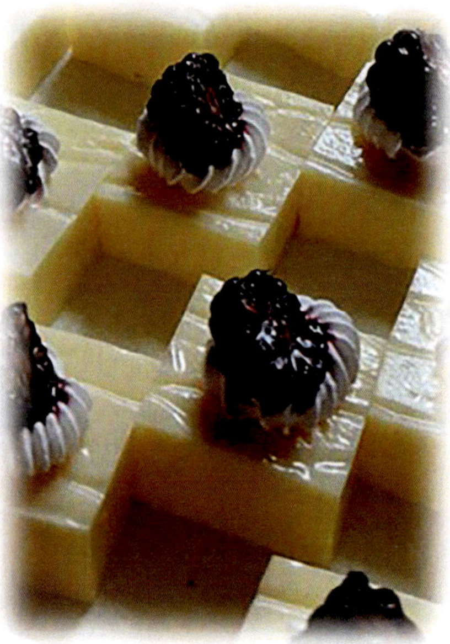

T-Shirt Thought

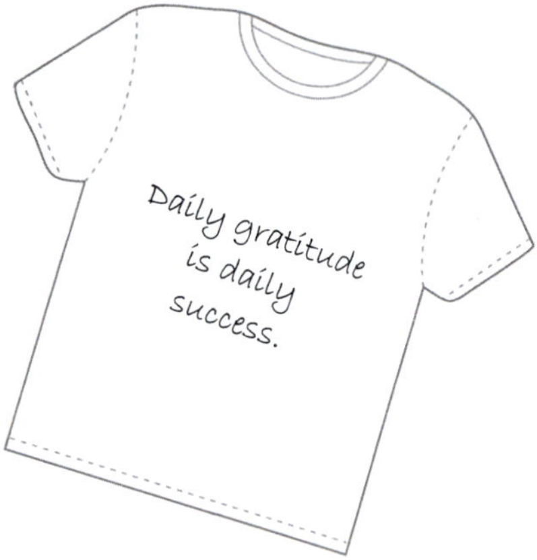

I am grateful; I am sympathetic

I am understanding; I am positive everyday

I am strong; I am dependable

I am honest; I am trustworthy

I will express my gratitude to the universe every day for all that I have and all that I am.

End of Day

Be grateful for all that you are.

CONTEMPLATION

I am cared for; I am loved

I am intelligent; I am talented

I am accomplished; I am appreciated

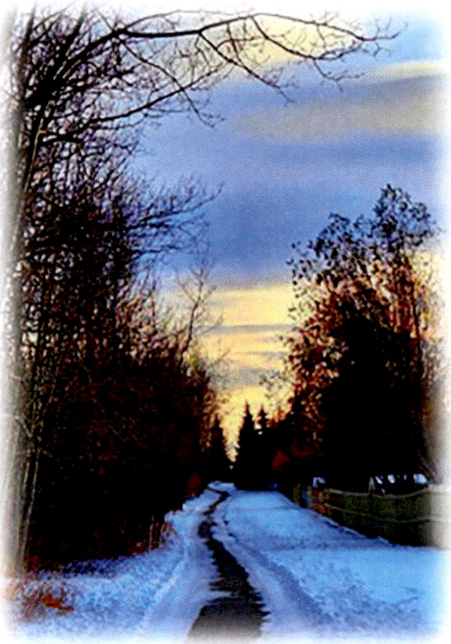

T-Shirt Thought

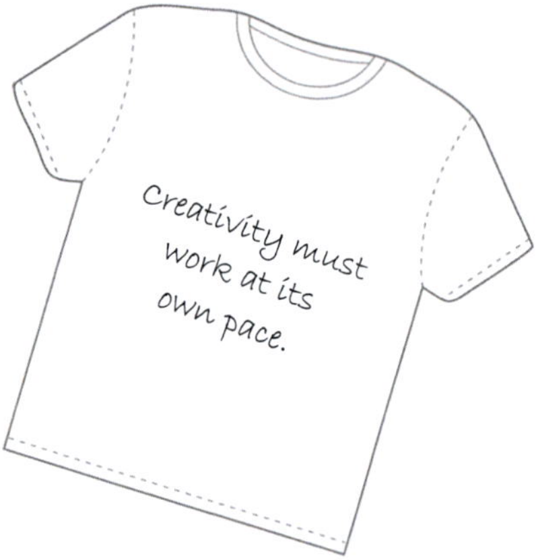

I am grateful; I am sympathetic

I am understanding; I am positive everyday

I am strong; I am dependable

I am honest; I am trustworthy

I will express my gratitude to the universe every day for all that I have and all that I am.

End of Day

When your body is telling you to rest, listen to it. It's taking care of your mind.

CONTEMPLATION

I am cared for; I am loved

I am intelligent; I am talented

I am accomplished; I am appreciated

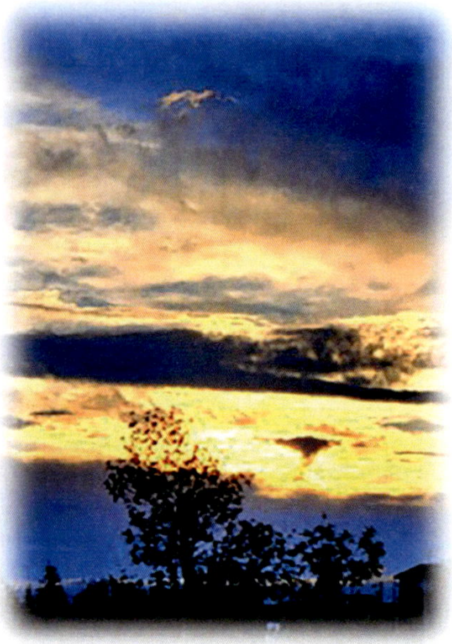

T-Shirt Thought

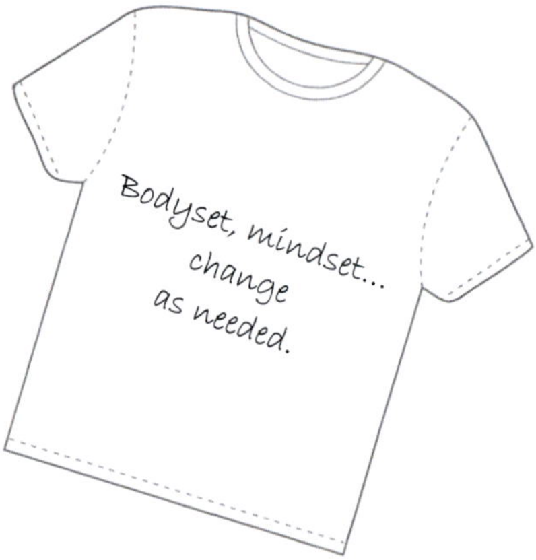

I am grateful; I am sympathetic

I am understanding; I am positive everyday

I am strong; I am dependable

I am honest; I am trustworthy

I will express my gratitude to the universe every day for all that I have and all that I am.

End of Day

When you realize you need an attitude change, you've already done half the work.

CONTEMPLATION

TOGETHER ON THE PATH

I am cared for; I am loved

I am intelligent; I am talented

I am accomplished; I am appreciated

T-Shirt Thought

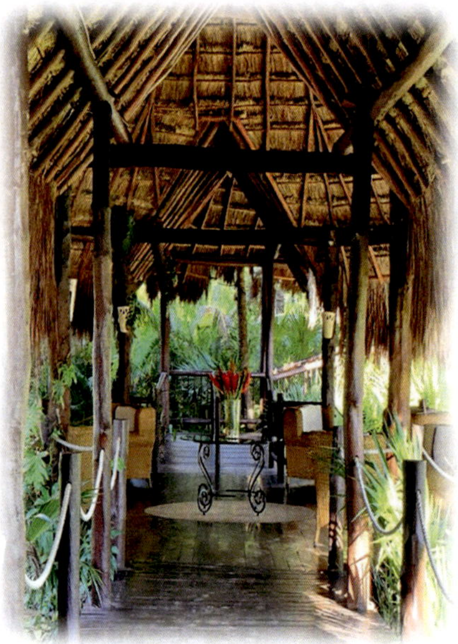

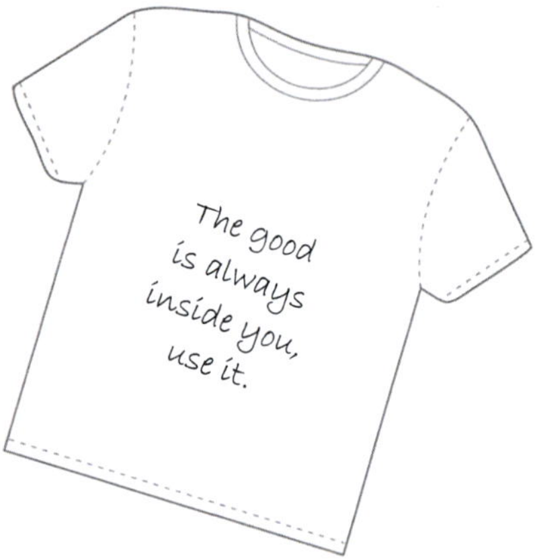

I am grateful; I am sympathetic

I am understanding; I am positive everyday

I am strong; I am dependable

I am honest; I am trustworthy

I will express my gratitude to the universe every day for all that I have and all that I am.

End of Day

When faced with a big decision, trust yourself. You know what's right for you.

CONTEMPLATION

I am cared for; I am loved

I am intelligent; I am talented

I am accomplished; I am appreciated

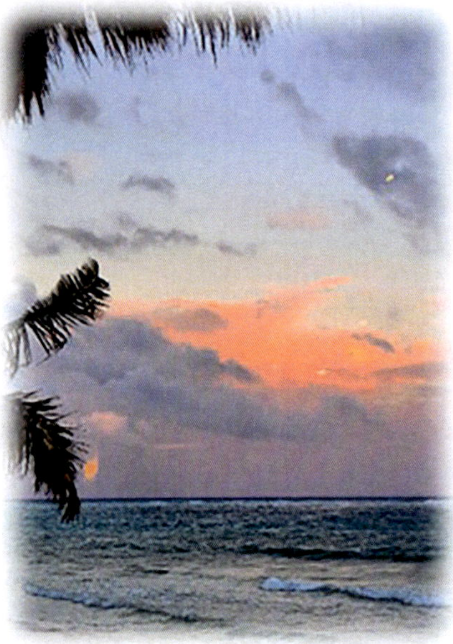

T-Shirt Thought

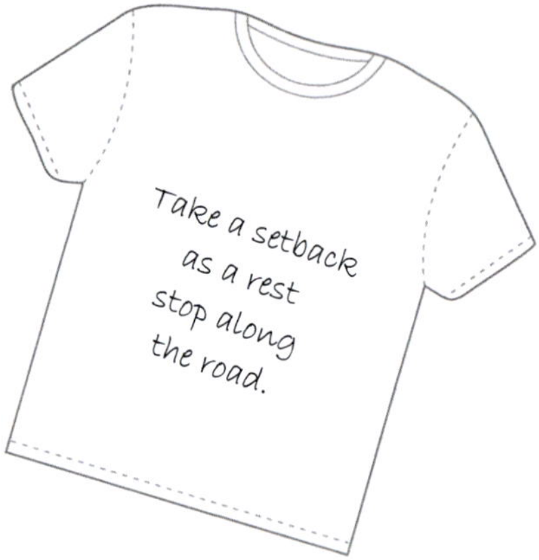

I am grateful; I am sympathetic

I am understanding; I am positive everyday

I am strong; I am dependable

I am honest; I am trustworthy

I will express my gratitude to the universe every day for all that I have and all that I am.

End of Day

Don't let disappointment spoil your day. Just re-arrange your perspective.

CONTEMPLATION

TOGETHER ON THE PATH

I am cared for; I am loved

I am intelligent; I am talented

I am accomplished; I am appreciated

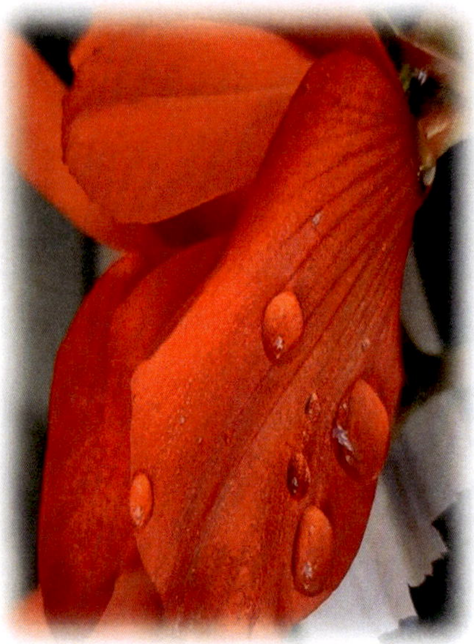

T-Shirt Thought

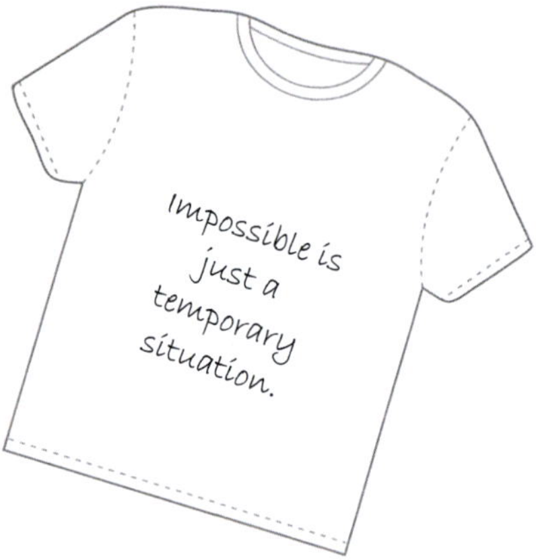

I am grateful; I am sympathetic

I am understanding; I am positive everyday

I am strong; I am dependable

I am honest; I am trustworthy

I will express my gratitude to the universe every day for all that I have and all that I am.

End of Day

When you tackle a problem with all that you are, that problem doesn't stand a chance.

CONTEMPLATION

I am cared for; I am loved

I am intelligent; I am talented

I am accomplished; I am appreciated

T-Shirt Thought

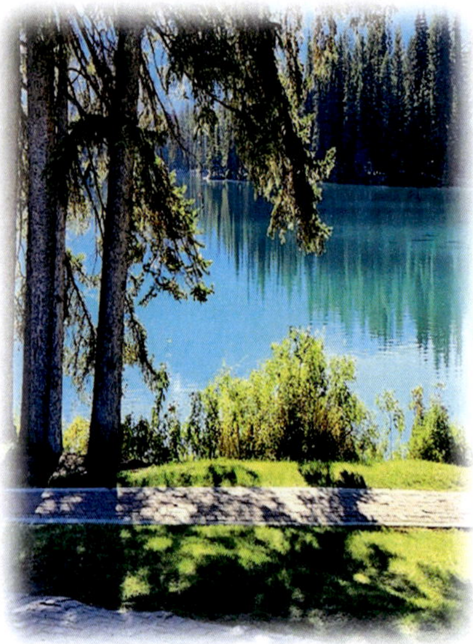

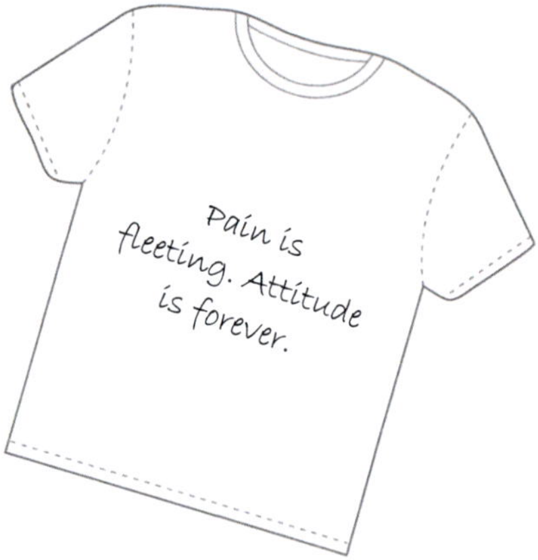

I am grateful; I am sympathetic

I am understanding; I am positive everyday

I am strong; I am dependable

I am honest; I am trustworthy

I will express my gratitude to the universe every day for all that I have and all that I am.

End of Day

Physical activity to the point of near exhaustion is so very satisfying every time.

CONTEMPLATION

I am cared for; I am loved

I am intelligent; I am talented

I am accomplished; I am appreciated

T-Shirt Thought

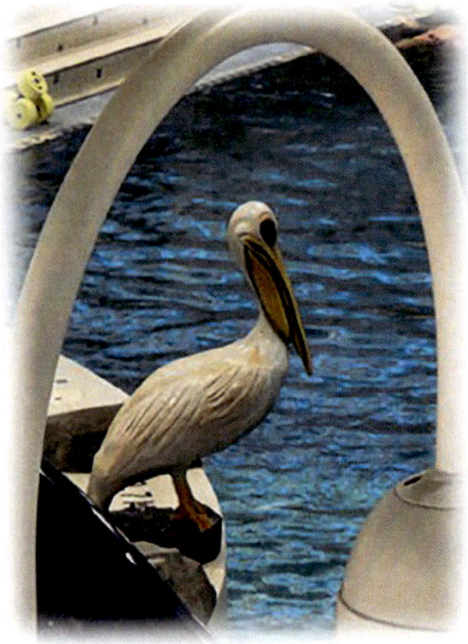

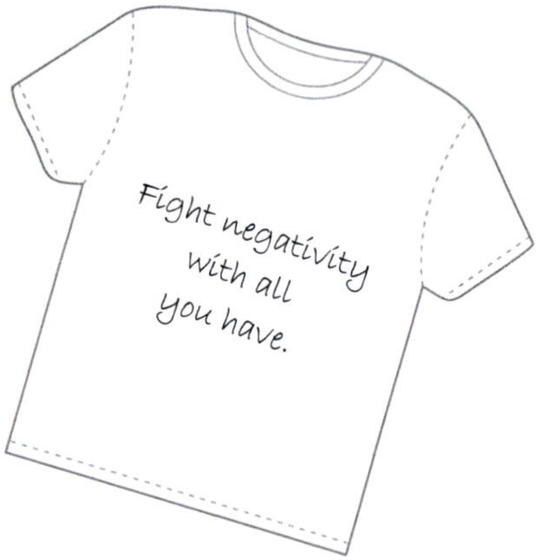

I am grateful; I am sympathetic

I am understanding; I am positive everyday

I am strong; I am dependable

I am honest; I am trustworthy

I will express my gratitude to the universe every day for all that I have and all that I am.

End of Day

When your day is overwhelming, stop, take a deep breath, and smile.

CONTEMPLATION

I am cared for; I am loved

I am intelligent; I am talented

I am accomplished; I am appreciated

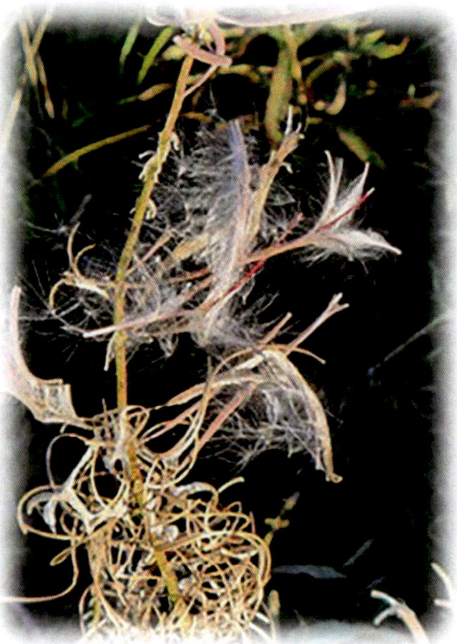

T-Shirt Thought

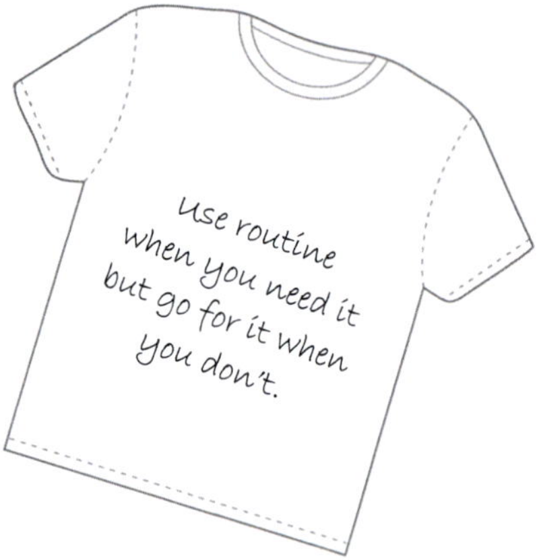

I am grateful; I am sympathetic

I am understanding; I am positive everyday

I am strong; I am dependable

I am honest; I am trustworthy

I will express my gratitude to the universe every day for all that I have and all that I am.

End of Day

If the day seems chaotic, look at it from inside yourself. You will see that it is exciting fun and motivating.

CONTEMPLATION

I am cared for; I am loved

I am intelligent; I am talented

I am accomplished; I am appreciated

T-Shirt Thought

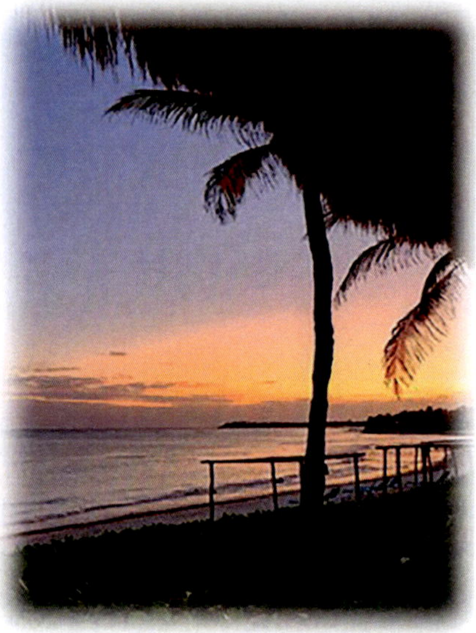

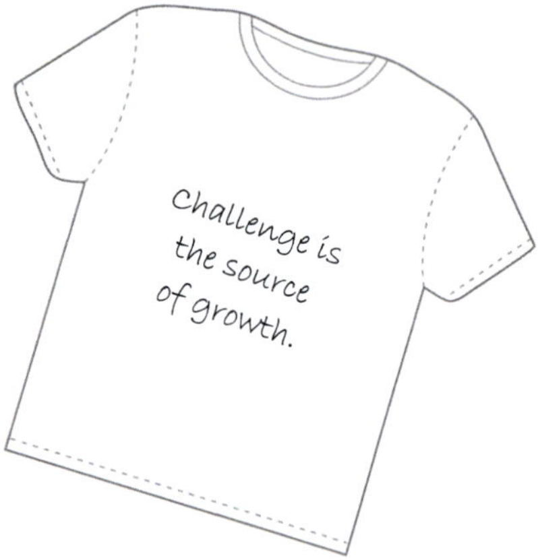

I am grateful; I am sympathetic

I am understanding; I am positive everyday

I am strong; I am dependable

I am honest; I am trustworthy

I will express my gratitude to the universe every day for all that I have and all that I am.

End of Day

Success is not only the accomplishment, it's the effort.

CONTEMPLATION

TOGETHER ON THE PATH

I am cared for; I am loved

I am intelligent; I am talented

I am accomplished; I am appreciated

T-Shirt Thought

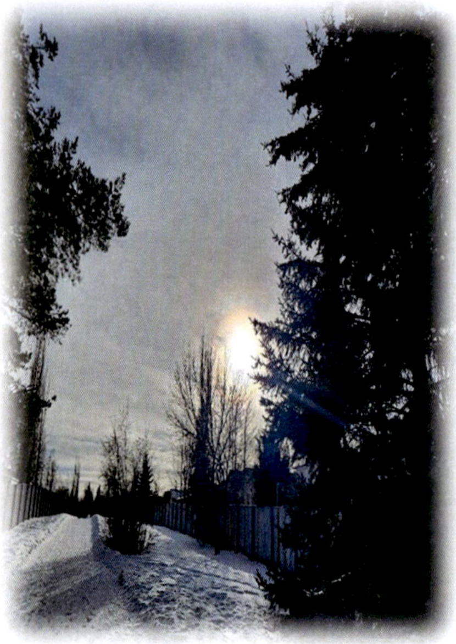

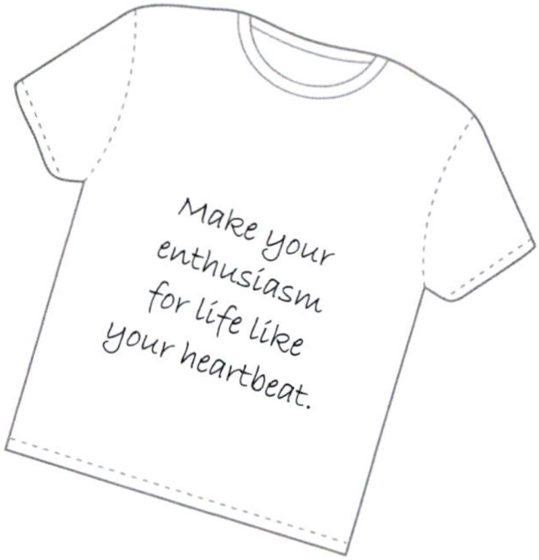

I am grateful; I am sympathetic

I am understanding; I am positive everyday

I am strong; I am dependable

I am honest; I am trustworthy

I will express my gratitude to the universe every day for all that I have and all that I am.

End of Day

If you play sports fairly and respectfully, you live fairly and respectfully.

CONTEMPLATION

I am cared for; I am loved

I am intelligent; I am talented

I am accomplished; I am appreciated

T-Shirt Thought

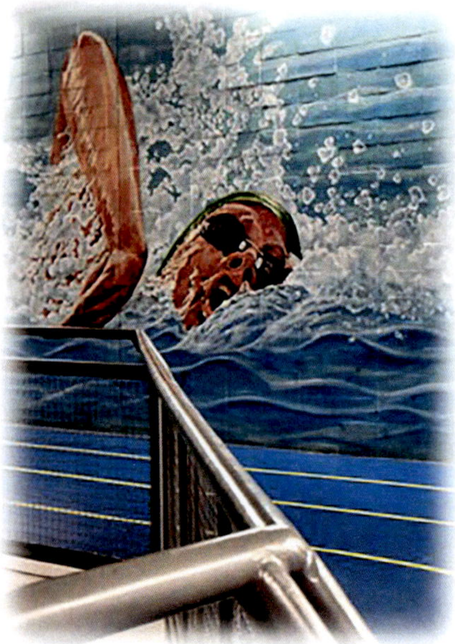

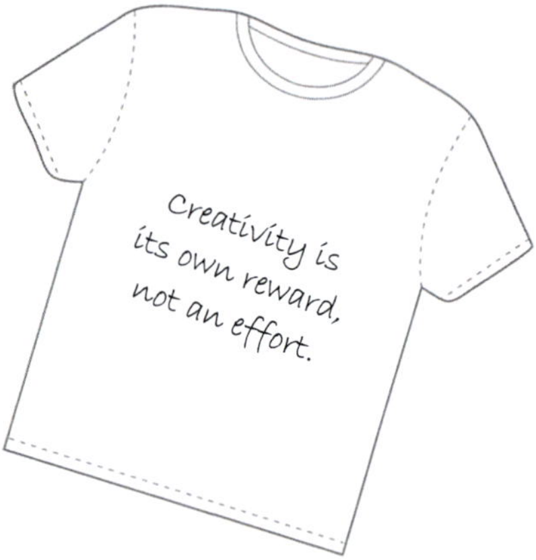

I am grateful; I am sympathetic

I am understanding; I am positive everyday

I am strong; I am dependable

I am honest; I am trustworthy

I will express my gratitude to the universe every day for all that I have and all that I am.

End of Day

Any interest can become a passion if we just let it.

CONTEMPLATION

I am cared for; I am loved

I am intelligent; I am talented

I am accomplished; I am appreciated

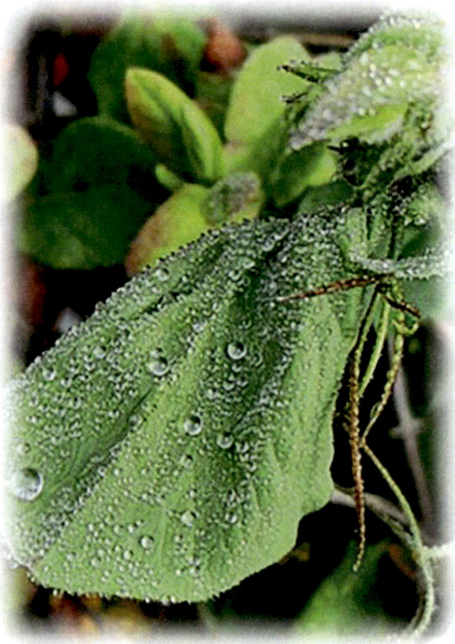

T-Shirt Thought

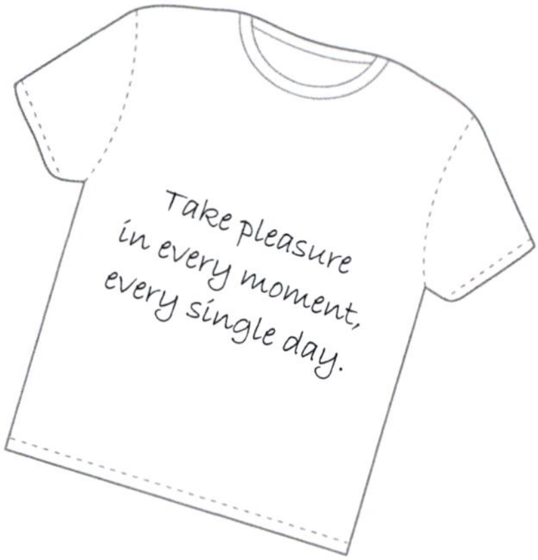

I am grateful; I am sympathetic

I am understanding; I am positive everyday

I am strong; I am dependable

I am honest; I am trustworthy

I will express my gratitude to the universe every day for all that I have and all that I am.

End of Day

Our attitudes can be changed with so little effort. Why not lean towards the positive every day?

CONTEMPLATION

I am cared for; I am loved

I am intelligent; I am talented

I am accomplished; I am appreciated

T-Shirt Thought

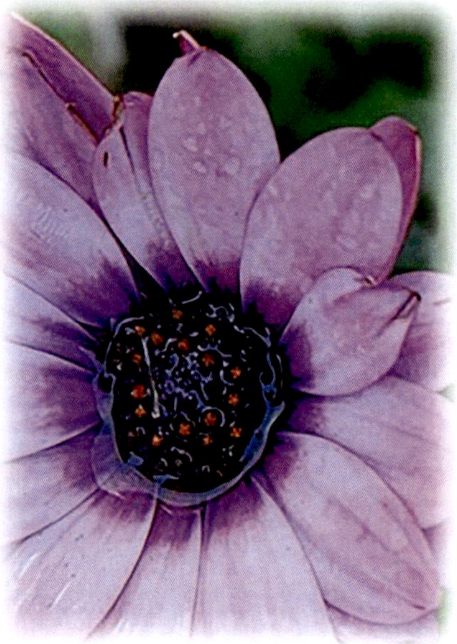

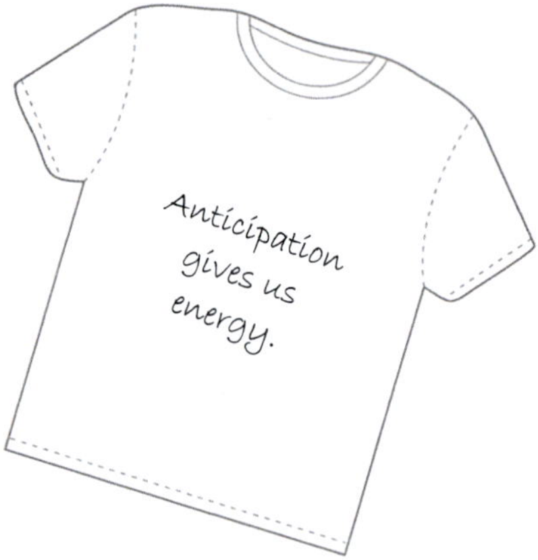

I am grateful; I am sympathetic

I am understanding; I am positive everyday

I am strong; I am dependable

I am honest; I am trustworthy

I will express my gratitude to the universe every day for all that I have and all that I am.

End of Day

Anticipation can be the sweetest kind of tension.

CONTEMPLATION

TOGETHER ON THE PATH

I am cared for; I am loved

I am intelligent; I am talented

I am accomplished; I am appreciated

T-Shirt Thought

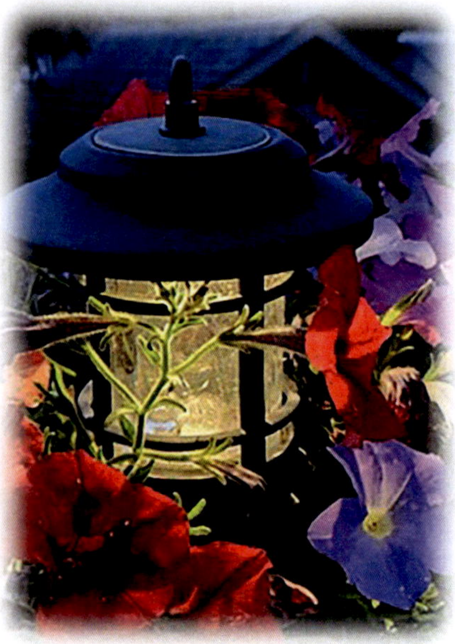

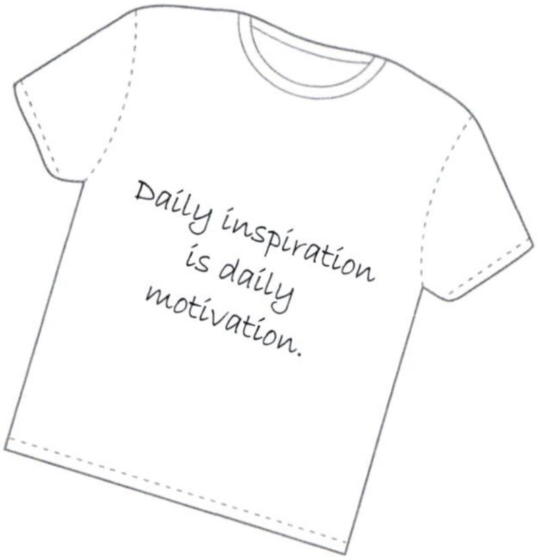

I am grateful; I am sympathetic

I am understanding; I am positive everyday

I am strong; I am dependable

I am honest; I am trustworthy

I will express my gratitude to the universe every day for all that I have and all that I am.

End of Day

Perseverance with confidence means success and satisfaction every time.

CONTEMPLATION

TOGETHER ON THE PATH

I am cared for; I am loved

I am intelligent; I am talented

I am accomplished; I am appreciated

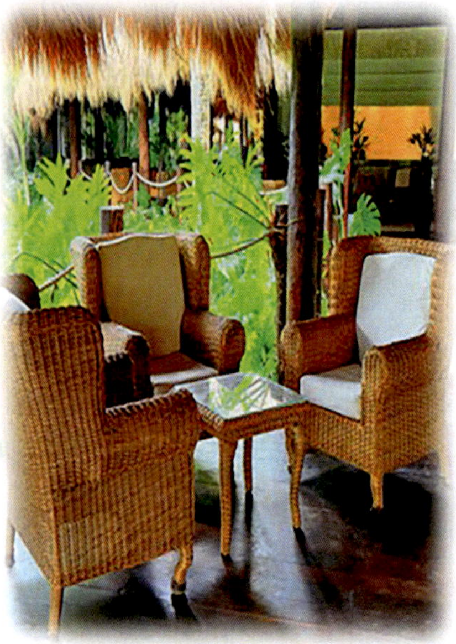

T-Shirt Thought

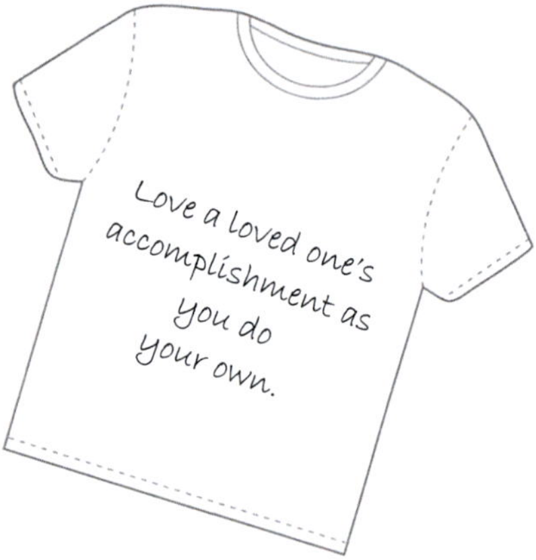

I am grateful; I am sympathetic

I am understanding; I am positive everyday

I am strong; I am dependable

I am honest; I am trustworthy

I will express my gratitude to the universe every day for all that I have and all that I am.

End of Day

It is so satisfying to see the success of others because of your influence.

CONTEMPLATION

TOGETHER ON THE PATH

I am cared for; I am loved

I am intelligent; I am talented

I am accomplished; I am appreciated

T-Shirt Thought

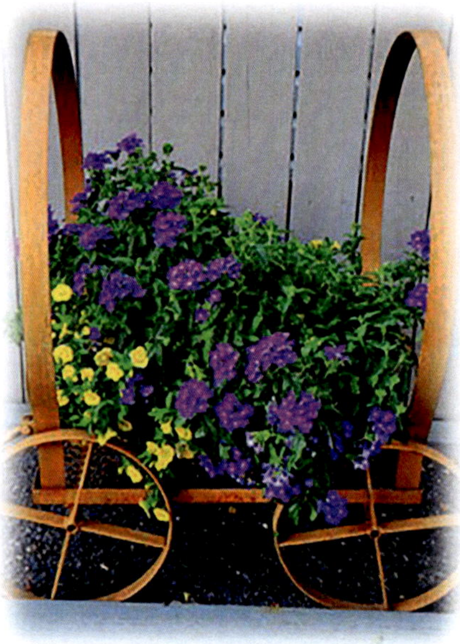

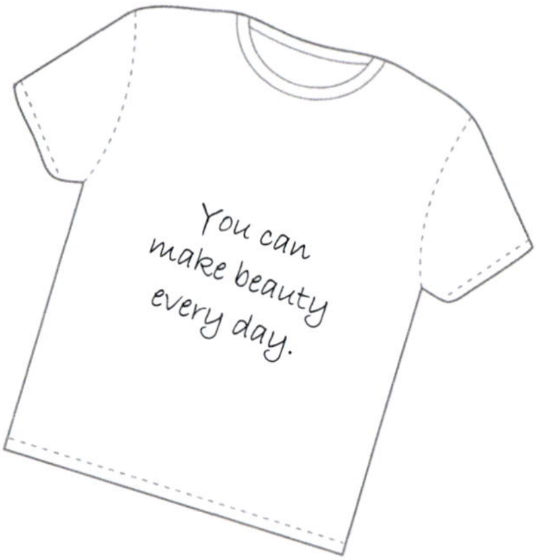

I am grateful; I am sympathetic

I am understanding; I am positive everyday

I am strong; I am dependable

I am honest; I am trustworthy

I will express my gratitude to the universe every day for all that I have and all that I am.

End of Day

Do something that soothes your soul every single day.

CONTEMPLATION

I am cared for; I am loved

I am intelligent; I am talented

I am accomplished; I am appreciated

T-Shirt Thought

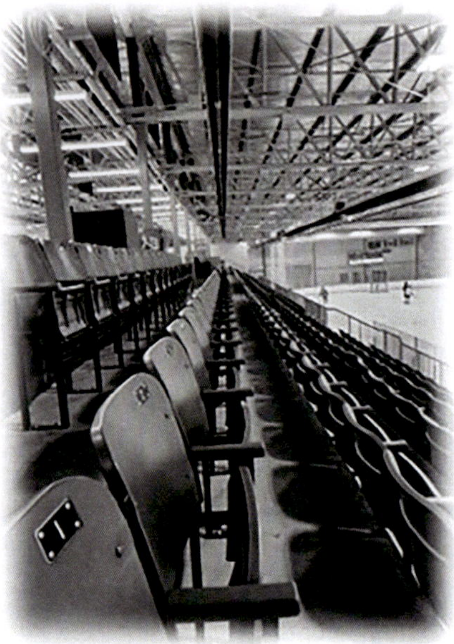

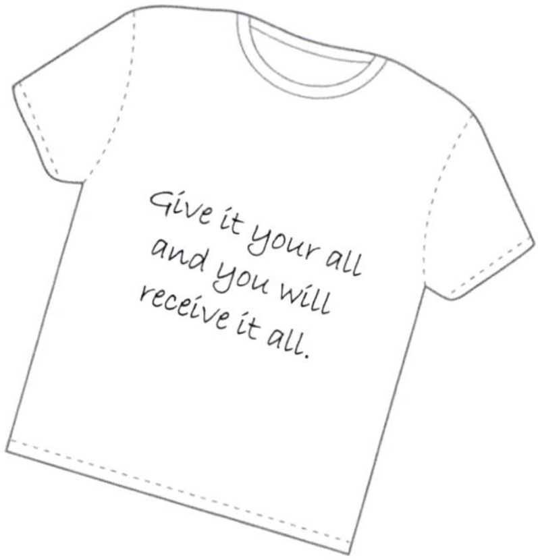

I am grateful; I am sympathetic

I am understanding; I am positive everyday

I am strong; I am dependable

I am honest; I am trustworthy

I will express my gratitude to the universe every day for all that I have and all that I am.

End of Day

A stressful day is not a wasted day.

CONTEMPLATION

I am cared for; I am loved

I am intelligent; I am talented

I am accomplished; I am appreciated

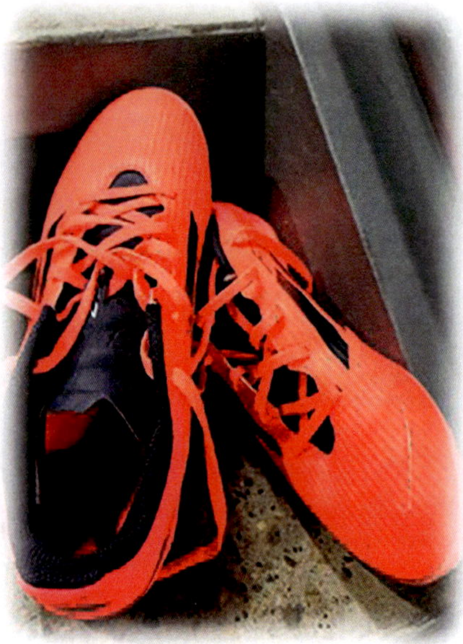

T-Shirt Thought

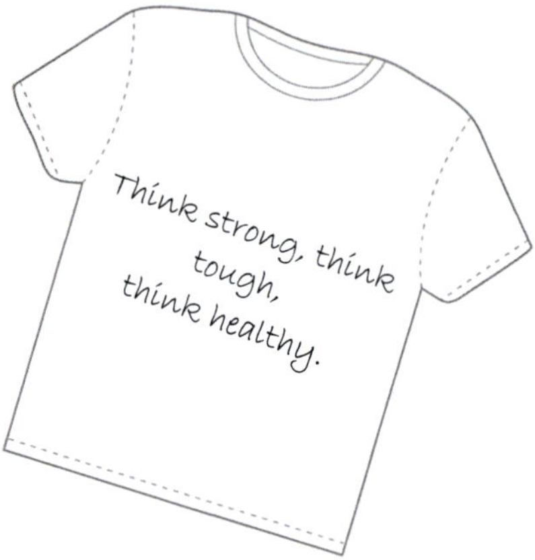

I am grateful; I am sympathetic

I am understanding; I am positive everyday

I am strong; I am dependable

I am honest; I am trustworthy

I will express my gratitude to the universe every day for all that I have and all that I am.

End of Day

The best way to influence people is to polish up your attitude.

CONTEMPLATION

I am cared for; I am loved

I am intelligent; I am talented

I am accomplished; I am appreciated

T-Shirt Thought

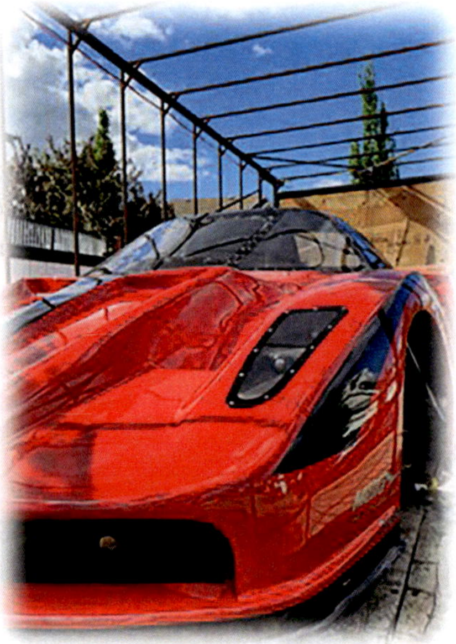

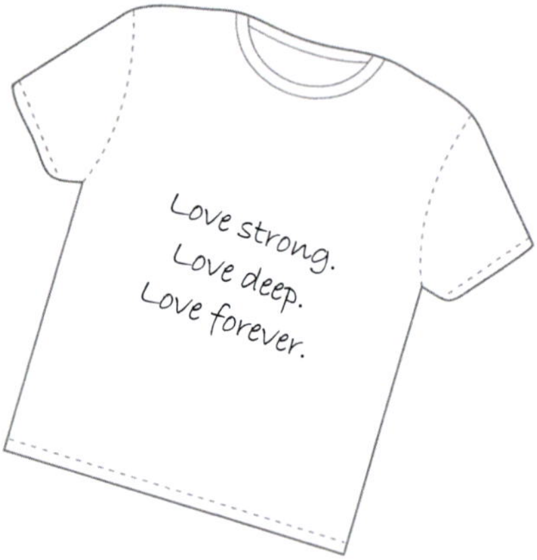

I am grateful; I am sympathetic

I am understanding; I am positive everyday

I am strong; I am dependable

I am honest; I am trustworthy

I will express my gratitude to the universe every day for all that I have and all that I am.

End of Day

Appreciate every single day, whether full of challenges or full of peace.

CONTEMPLATION

Summary

We have now completed this leg of our journey and once again we have learned more about ourselves; our strengths and our determination to become more positive, more confident and so much more appreciative of all that we have and all that we are.

This is a huge success and a truly worthwhile endeavor.